TALK TO YOUR BODY

RETHINKING HEALING
BY
RETHINKING REALITY

BY BEN MOSES

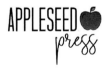

Talk to Your Body: Rethinking Healing by Rethinking Reality

Copyright © 2002 by Ben Moses.
Second Edition Copyright © 2017 by Ben Moses.

Published by Appleseed Press
Los Angeles, California

All Rights Reserved. Except as permitted under the United States Copyright Act of 1976, no part of this publication may be reproduced or distributed in any form or by any means, or stored in a data base or retrieval system, without the prior written permission of the author, except in the case of brief quotations embodied in critical articles and reviews.

2023

> *In all these years I'll bet you've never left your exalted perch behind the big windows to slide down your medulla oblongata and say hello to the tireless workers whose job it is to hold your head erect.*
>
> *It's time to change that.*

Dear Susie,

A dear friend is author. Hope you find his words/ideas helpful.

Merry, merry,
Charlotte

For Lynne, who daily teaches me
more about living
than I ever thought there was to know.

Ben Moses, Emmy-winning documentarian, filmmaker, musician and TV/radio engineer, was born into a Midwestern family of Pentecostal church-goers who considered faith healing and speaking in tongues a part of God's gift to true believers.

Thus the stage was set for his life-long interest in how healing works. Witnessing amazing healings but believing this ability couldn't be the exclusive province of that tiny religion, Ben set out to uncover how healing works, and how he could apply it without all the trappings. Then he experienced his own "impossible" healing, and set about to develop a way to apply the process in daily life, with injuries and illnesses that otherwise might be serious or debilitating.

"Talk to Your Body" helps remove the fear that disease or injury (or even death) can strike at any time and there's nothing you can do about it. The fear we feel because we seem to have no control over – and certainly no communication with – our body and its state of health.

In this book Ben shares his powerful journey toward this simple, seemingly revolutionary healing process that can change how you approach your body, your health and your life – without the mystical, metaphysical or religious requirements non-medical healing approaches are too often packaged with – and shows you how to use them, alone, or with your doctor or medical practitioner.

NOTICE TO THE READER

The information contained herein is not a substitute for diagnosis and treatment by a qualified, licensed professional. It is offered to the reader solely as a method of self-help to be used as an adjunct to, not a substitute for, appropriate professional help.

The author does not imply or encourage that the reader should apply these techniques in any specific instance of illness or injury or in lieu of obtaining proper and timely medical attention.

CONTENTS

PREFACE		i
Chapter I:	Allowing Possibilities	1
Chapter II:	Conversations with a Mole	13
Chapter III:	Altering States	25
Chapter IV:	The Other Half of Reality	35
Chapter V:	Intention: Our Fundamental Reality	46
Chapter VI:	The Great I AM	52
Chapter VII:	What If? Making New Metaphors	74
Chapter VIII:	Into the Depths of Fear	85
Chapter IX:	Acting on Your Belief	95
Chapter X:	Look What You Did to Me!	102
Chapter XI:	Finding Your Own Path	109
Chapter XII:	Take Your Healing Where You Find It	120
Chapter XIII:	Out of the Closet	128
Chapter XIV:	Talk to Your Body About Your Death	136
Chapter XV:	Now It's Your Turn	138
Epilogue:	Working With The Doctor	142
APPENDIX		161

PREFACE

When I was a child, faith healing, the classic evangelical, Deep South "holy roller" kind, was as natural to me as eating pork chops with your fingers. I was raised in a Pentecostal church in a small town in the Midwest. My mother was a born-again Christian before it was fashionable, and my father was from Louisiana – Deep South, evangelical Praise-the-Lord Louisiana.

Before I knew how to hold a fork I was exposed to Sunday healing services and summer tent revival meetings. I was prayed over at two when I had whooping cough, at four with pneumonia, and the summer I was eight I remember our portly pastor's sweat dripping on me as he bent over my sickbed entreating God to heal me from asthma. A few months later the long-haired cat who slept on my pillow got run over by a car, and those fervent prayers were finally answered. God works in mysterious ways.

On family vacations across the South we'd drive hundreds of miles out of our way to attend services featuring one or another firebrand preacher who practiced the art of laying on of hands. The performance was always part Messenger of God, part P.T. Barnum. To paraphrase Barnum, there's a hypochondriac born every minute. My mother was a hypochondriac, her mother was a hypochondriac, and my father, bless his soul, was longsuffering. But just because you're a hypochondriac doesn't mean "Disease" isn't out to get you.

In my grandmother's case, the healings never seemed to last. A few weeks after a miraculous recovery she'd be down with something new, searching for another Reverend Billy Joe Bob on the gospel stump ready to once again invoke the *POW-ER!* (emphasis on "Pow"). Her belief that God could heal her was in the same category as smokers who believe they can quit – because He'd done it so many times before. It was the concept of permanence she had trouble with. Dad always just figured she enjoyed the spectacle and special attention of the process more than she enjoyed good health. As for me, I watched it all with a child's wide-eyed wonder, believing whatever the grownups believed, without question...for a while.

In spite of those like my grandmother who suffered in constant need of curing, I learned that many times in these services something unusual *was* going on – people with real diseases were in fact being healed. After all, how could the guy up on the stage show his face for long if it weren't so? You'd think after awhile anyone's bound to run out of hypochondriacs.

By the time I was 18 and off to college, I had witnessed scores of such healings, and knew people who walked away freed of colds and crutches...and cancer. But I couldn't accept the idea that this could only happen in the context of our particular religious belief. I couldn't believe God would only give this gift to a few thousand souls in this small sub-set of American Protestantism and to no one else. So by 18 I had departed the faith of my childhood, set on a quest to find out why and how that amazing healing process I had so often witnessed really worked, and if everyone could access that power – without the Pow.

As luck (or Providence) would have it, my first college roommate was a senior year philosophy major. He introduced me to the collection of 30 "Great Books of the Western World," and soon the writings of Aristotle, Plato, and Thomas Aquinas became my bedside companions, rather than the engineering textbooks I had a scholarship to study.

Over the next years, in between learning Boyle's law and calculating capacitive reactance in a tuned circuit, I read with fascination of the work of Edgar Cayce (the "sleeping prophet," as a biographer dubbed him), the work of the Caddys and Dorothy Maclean at Findhorn[1] and the musings of metaphysical minds like

---

[1] The Findhorn spiritual community, founded in Morayshire, Scotland in 1962, established a vegetable garden in barren, rocky soil, which became known

Besant, Blavatsky, Jung, and Swedenborg, to name a few. Years later I met the teachings of Ernest Holmes, Krishnamurti and Rudolf Steiner. Each new thought, every new piece of information forced me to open my mind a bit more, allowing my concept of what was possible in the universe to expand ever so slightly.

I moved to New York City in the '70s, where I worked in television to pay the rent and in my free time found myself haunting the bookstores for more of this esoteric knowledge. Having read the Bible through a couple times in my youth, now, in the vast melting pot of cultures that is New York, I met followers of Buddha, Krishna, Mohammed, believers in Joseph Smith, Siddartha, Seth[2], Satayananda and probably the Man in the Moon for all I can remember. At the urging of these sages I had many sleepless nights reading the Rig Veda, the Bhagavad Gita, the Koran, and, in some Indiana motel during a long location shoot, the Book of Mormon.

I debated philosophy and reality with friends in robes and sandals who chanted on the streets, with Tarot card and tea leaf readers, with some who smoked weed for a living, still others who slept under pyramids, mirrors, purple light, swore by E-meters,[3] believed they came from distant planets or channeled one or another supposed entity, known or unknown.

Usually motivated more by my desire to be in the company of some beautiful woman than by any interest in her religion, I sat in meditation at the Zen Center, had my engrams assessed at Scientology, learned the ways of the Great Spirit in a Native American sweat lodge[4], and heard first-hand accounts of medicine men using raw steaks and cryptic incantations to draw out and heal deep infections. From Hindu texts I learned of a special holy

---

worldwide for its unprecedented abundance and outrageously large produce. See www.findhorn.org

[2] A higher dimensional "Energy essence personality" purportedly channeled by Jane Roberts. See "Seth Speaks" and other books by Roberts

[3] Psychological testing device used in Scientology

[4] Traditional Native American spiritual ritual

water drunk by devotees of yore that permitted you to see God; LSD users told me they were getting the same results from a little sugar cube. From Cajun seers I heard of poultices that could cure gout and suck tumors through the skin.

But whatever my reason for being there, each experience left me with new information and often a profound appreciation for yet another way of reaching out to the Infinite. By the time I left New York I was pouring through Gurgieff and Goethe and had joined the Association for Research and Enlightenment (the Edgar Cayce foundation) to learn more about this amazing man.

In Los Angeles I found more interesting healing ceremonies, most conducted with intricate theatrics, which I came to believe were designed, consciously or unconsciously, to alter the patient's psyche and permit healing where none could take hold before, just like the Pentecostal practitioners of my youth.

Some of what I have witnessed has been called sorcery, superstition and witchcraft, some in the past have burned books about it, or even the practitioners themselves, but I have learned that in spite of the beliefs of the burners, the observers or even the recipients, healing can happen, in the most curious times and places.

While all this was fascinating to me, for years it remained in the realm of "who knows what's real and what's not?" as I went about the business of my life. It wasn't until I starting thinking about it in the context of my engineering and science background that it began to come together. From college I had learned about quantum physics, about Heisenberg[5] and the *uncertainty* principal, the *probability* theory, Einstein's two *relativities* (*general* and *special*), and the postulate that the observer influences the experiment. I loved the anthropic principal, the idea that it's only our observation of the universe that makes it real. Then I entertained

---

[5] Werner Heisenberg (1901-1976) is the father of quantum mechanics.

Schrödinger's cat[6] in the box for awhile, and became gradually fascinated with the seemingly obvious correlation between religion, mystical metaphysics, and what new physics was saying about the non-reality that underpins our wonderfully simple everyday concept of reality.

Observing the increasing overlaps of those two disparate practices, science and religion, I began to get a glimmer that possibly faith healing might have a scientific explanation after all – and if it had that, then it could be repeated, for science is founded on the repeatability of the experiment.

But this was still all quite theoretical; it would be years before I experimented with it in my own life. When I finally did, I was so astonished at the results that I kept it secret from all but my closest friends, for fear people would think I was crazy.

Clearly there are as many varieties of healing techniques as there are people who wish to be healed. And people are often healed by many of these arcane techniques – especially if their illnesses are not too serious, or not too far along, and most especially if they participate in the process with their whole being.

But there seems to be one thing common to all forms of healing: It is evident that if, like my grandmother, one cannot completely adjust to the new lease on life their healing has given them, then it will not last; their predisposition to be ill will ultimately overpower any cure offered by medical doctor or medicine man.

---

[6] Austrian physicist Erwin Schroedinger postulated that an atom can be in two different states at once, decayed and undecayed. Only when an observer actually tries to determine the state of the atom does the atom assume one of the states. Therefore, a cat in a closed box can be both dead and alive; it only assumes one state or the other when you open the box.

Too, there seems to be something special and simple that sages of medicine and health have overlooked. The Bible gives us a foundation for it and modern science's understanding of our true reality proves that it is possible. Call it creating an imaginary anthropomorphic *gestalt* from unintelligent cells and organs; call it conceiving of your body as a clustering of related and sentient parts you can address directly and consciously; call it *talking to your body*. It is the subject of this book.

Over the years, I have learned how to help – how to allow – my body to heal, just like the fire and brimstone healers of my youth, often in apparently miraculous ways, but without the pretense, the sleight-of-hand, the incantations and theatrics used by many, and without the specific religious structure imposed on it by the well-intentioned folk I grew up with.

I'm not perfect at it, I never will be. Death will eventually catch me, I'm sure. But it has helped me stay unusually healthy and vibrant through the last 30 years, when many of my peers – all of us barking at 70's door – are beginning to experience the onset of serious and debilitating illness.

I want to pass the word around, because I know that, as well as it works for me, there will be others who will be more successful at using this process than I. I hope that as others – even you, perhaps – begin to experiment with this novel, simple way of approaching healing, we may all hear of your own success with it. That will encourage the rest of us to try again, with greater assurance. And after a while, this almost impossible-to-believe magic will take its place among the mundane techniques of healing, and we will have succeeded in ripping away yet another veil from the superstition and ignorance that surrounds our knowledge of ourselves. Remember, it wasn't that many years ago that cultured bread mold[7] became a miracle cure, and today it is passé.

---

[7] Common penicillin

To be sure, I do not for a moment suggest that if you are sick all you do is talk to your body. Too many wise and intelligent people, Western and Eastern, mystical, allopathic and alternative healers, have studied the human physical condition for too many centuries to just ignore this accumulated knowledge. Personally, I like big pharmaceutical companies' antibiotics for infections, combined with a healthy dose of (double Nobel laureate) Dr. Linus Pauling's favorite chemical, Vitamin C, and water and orange juice and rest…AND a conversation with my body about what's going on and what we can do together to set things right. Then we "create possibility."

One key to understanding my approach is this: the commonly used term "physical health" implies that there is some meaningful separation between our physical-ness and the other aspects of "us," our spiritual- and mental- "nesses." But I have come to realize there is not. When the physical is treated, the spiritual and mental are affected, *and vice versa*. We are whole beings, *aspects* of which can be described in many varied ways by scholars or observers, depending solely on how they choose to look at us, or more to the point, where they choose to stop looking.

In that regard, the concept of the Trinity has always fascinated me, as if someone big has been trying to tell us about the unity of three beings in one for a long time now, but our ancestors never quite got it. Can a Christian believer defy the Father, but the Son and the Holy Spirit "don't notice?" Of course not. Neither can you alter your mental state without your physical and spiritual states being affected.

In fact the line between spiritual and physical or mental is ultimately an arbitrary one, drawn centuries ago, from ignorance, for the convenience of the observer, teacher, student and practitioner, and maintained still today as an academic convention, having less and less meaning to us.

Somewhere inside us we really understand this, which is why it is sometimes difficult to accept treatment from someone who sees only the "piece of meat" aspect of us while ignoring the rest. But the doctor who works on the piece of meat often has a lot of ability to help your body heal, and I recommend using every tool in the toolbox when the time comes.

I hope this book will give you another big tool for your box. Use it early and often, and you may be surprised, as I still am every time, at how well it does the job.

Ben Moses
Los Angeles 2017

*"Each patient carries his own doctor inside him.
They come to us not knowing that truth."*

-- Dr. Albert Schweitzer

As quoted by Norman Cousins in
Anatomy of an Illness as Perceived by the Patient
(New York: W. W. Norton, 2005), paperback ed., 78.

Chapter I: Allowing Possibilities

Imagine you're an oarsman on a small ship in the king's navy. Port side, sixteenth row, middle seat. One ship of a hundred, or a thousand, you don't know, and have no way of ever finding out, even if you could think the question, which you cannot. Your brain isn't big enough for that.

You were born to do this, as were your parents before you. You don't remember not being here, not doing this. You don't mind, because you can't think to mind. You're not a slave, you're perfectly in your element, your entire existence is for that one thing only: moving your oar in concert with the hundreds of others around you, and if you feel joy, you feel it most when you are rowing full out. That's your function, and you do it perfectly.

There is a Captain of your ship, a powerful, all-knowing guide who takes care of everything in your existence. You know he was there in the beginning, and she resides on the bridge somewhere else in the ship, but he has never come to visit; she sends subordinates to handle all matters having to do with you.

As for the king whom your Captain serves, that may as well be God himself, you've never seen him, and never will.

For years now you have performed your function perfectly, and all is well. But one day at no particular time, for there is no time in your existence, something completely unknown happens; something terrible. From out of nowhere, so far as you can tell, a great force suddenly smashes into the ship, buckling the hull and the deck above, which come crashing down on you, immobilizing you. Water rushes in and covers you, then the ship rights itself, and all becomes still. The water recedes, and you try to row again, but you cannot. You are filled with pain, and terrified. You have no idea what has happened, you are ignorant of anything ever like this. A signal is transmitted to the bridge, alerting the captain to the damaged area. You wait, immobilized and in shock.

A rescue team arrives and boards up the hull and deck, but you are in pain now, not capable of rowing normally; you can hardly breathe. Paramedics come on the scene, check you over for damage and begin the rudiments of repair. You reach out to them for more, for answers, but they are like you, only there to do their job.

Knowing nothing else to do, you attempt to return to the security of your routine, automatically going through the motions of rowing, but you still cannot. It will take time to return to normal, the shock and terror of the experience will not wear off quickly. To help that you need emotional assistance now, and there is no one equipped to take care of you in that way.

But then a miracle occurs. The great and all-wise Captain appears beside you. She checks you over and tells you in her sure and certain way that you are fine, and healing quickly. He understands what you've been through, and is proud of you. She may even apologize for not having been to visit you before. He puts his hand on your shoulder and tells you just how important you are to the well-being of the ship, that everything is all right now, you've weathered the storm admirably, and all is well.

Upon hearing the comforting words of this powerful leader you trust, the fear leaves your body and you relax. As he stands with you, you know that everything's going to be okay. With this encouragement, you realize you can row again, and what pain you may have is not important anymore, because you understand now that it will subside. Because you trust the Captain completely, everything in your existence returns to normal quickly.

This works in the real world, in business, in the military, in the doctor's office, and in our national security. Remember how important it was after September 11th, 2001 for the President and the nation's leaders to assure us everything was all right. In a shocking, out of the ordinary situation, we all look to some authority we trust to tell us we're okay.

What we haven't realized is, it works that way in our bodies, too. Every cell, organ, muscle, bone, can be perceived as one of our ship's crew. Each is devoted to performing one perfect function, and when something unusual happens, they all look to the Captain of their ship to let them know they're okay. They don't have the brains to know what's next – that's the Brain's job, your job, as the Captain.

In this book you're going to learn how to be the captain of your own ship. The benevolent, all knowing God of your body's universe, and your body will thank you, because now, perhaps for the first time in its life, it has a leader it can look to in time of trouble.

Here's how it began for me:

In 1984, after exploring healing from the detached perspective of a "seeker of wisdom and truth" for a dozen years, my own experience with healing arrived and hit me hard in the face – right in the eye, to be specific. I woke up one morning with what looked like a spider web in my right eye. Not long before, a friend had almost lost his sight because of a detached retina, so I knew what spider web symptoms meant, and I was scared.

I was on a business trip in Atlanta, far from home, and it was a Sunday morning. I hadn't a clue as to what eye specialist I should see, but I knew I wanted to see one fast. I called a friend in New York, who worked in the field, and asked him for advice. He put me in touch with the head of the Emory University Eye Center. My friend said I was lucky to be in Atlanta, Emory was one of the best eye centers in the country.

When I described the symptoms to Emory's chief ophthalmologist on the phone, he told me to meet him in his office in 45 minutes – which of course shot my anxiety level sky high. This was a *Sunday*, after all! After dilating my eye and inspecting it thoroughly, he gave me the bad news: I had a *macular pucker* – a puckering of the retina – and it was irreversible. He said my vision in that eye would deteriorate over the next few months to severely limited or none. There was an invasive operation that could be done, in which they would slice into the eye from the side and cut away that part of the retina that was already puckered, then try to laser the remaining part back onto the posterior wall of the eye. But it was risky at best. Yikes.

Hearing that I taught at UCLA, he recommended I go to the university's Jules Stein Eye Center when I got home, and the next day he helped arrange an immediate appointment with one of the leading retina specialists there.

I was a mess; I cut my business short and headed home. On the plane I couldn't think of anything else. Wherever I looked, the spider web went with me. I expected at any moment to see the spider crawling into view. I was distraught, scared and frustrated. My favorite hobby was flying; how would I be able to fly with only one eye? I was too young. At a moment like this, no matter how old you are, you're too young.

At UCLA, the specialist put me through another battery of tests, then put away his tools and faced me with the facts: within five months I would lose the vision in my right eye. There was nothing they could do.

I couldn't believe it. I couldn't imagine that there was nothing this internationally renowned eye research center could do to prevent the loss of my vision. That was an unacceptable conclusion. I asked him what were my chances, in case he was wrong. He said two percent. In his years of practice, he had never seen anyone with my condition have anything more than light-dark vision after six months. I asked him about the operation the Emory ophthalmologist had discussed. He said it wouldn't help in my case.

A two percent chance to still be able to see with that eye in six months! I sat there numb. I thought about it for a moment and realized I had two choices. I took the better one. I got up from the chair, thanked him for his time, and said, "So you say it is possible it won't happen." He shrugged and shook his head slowly, understanding my grasping for some hope, however remote. Then I added, "I'm going to be that two percent guy."

He wished me luck, and said, "Let me know. I'd like to see you in six months if you're right." I walked straight out, not stopping to say goodbye. I was going to be Mister Two Percent. Why not me? Somebody had to.

The next night I attended a dinner party at the home of my friends Stephan and Hayden Schwartz. Stephan had worked under Chief of Naval Operations Admiral Elmo Zumwalt[8] in Washington in the '70s, studying the Soviet Union's use of Extra Sensory Perception (ESP) in naval applications. He became fascinated with the extent to which the Soviets attempted to develop and use ESP and other "paranormal" techniques in military operations.

Now in civilian life, Stephan was running The Mobius Group, the only non-governmental operation using scientific method to study psychic functioning, or "Psi" as those in the field called it. For several years he had conducted stringently controlled experiments with people who exhibited psychic tendencies, and hired out his team to do investigations for such organizations as Interpol. the FBI, and local and state police departments around the country. His experimental findings and the results of the highly successful investigations were published in various scientific journals, supported by letters from the police agencies and institutions involved confirming the results. The Mobius research was the only unclassified scientific work in the field for many

---

[8] Commander US Naval Forces in Vietnam, 1968-70, Chief of Naval Operations and member of the Joint Chiefs of Staff, 1971-75.

years.⁹ Suffice it to say, he and his team were doing fascinating, impossible things.

At the Schwartz's party I found the man I was looking for, Jack Houck, an astrophysicist in the secret "skunk works" of one of the large aerospace companies in Los Angeles...and also, in his free time, a student of *psi*, as well as firewalking and, my favorite, spoon bending – "psychokinesis" or "PK," as it is known.

Jack had become interested in the deformation of metal by the mind at about the same time Stephan had, from learning about the (not so) secret Soviet experiments during the '70s. And, of course, an Israeli psychic named Uri Gellar was a controversial guest on every television talk show in those days, demonstrating his amazing ability to make forks and spoons bend on command, stop watches from ticking, and other sideshow stunts illustrating the powers of the mind.

The interesting part of Gellar's demonstration was that no one ever believed he was really doing it – they kept looking for the strings, and finding none. No one, that is, except the CIA and the Army's top secret Delta Force, who both were experimenting in the field themselves. They figured if they could bend rifle barrels and tank snouts just the tiniest bit, they could disable an entire mechanized division without firing a shot. Of course the Soviets were thinking the same thing, and they, too, were hard at work on the challenge.

Jack Houck was first and foremost a physicist, a hard science guy, and he was determined to uncover exactly what happened when someone like Gellar caused metal to bend – and to replicate the process if possible. After serious investigation, he concluded it wasn't just a sleight-of-hand trick. He reduced the process to something he thought could be taught, and then began

---

⁹ For more on the Mobius work, read *The Alexandria Project*, by Stephan A. Schwartz, and *Second Sight*, by Dr. Judith Orloff

to teach, starting his own weekend "PK evenings," better known to most of his friends as "spoon bending parties."

Anyone who brought silverware could join in the evenings, and Jack would lead them through the fascinating process of first focusing their minds and then yelling at their silverware to bend. It reminded me of the "*He*-Yal!" demand made by the Pentecostal healers of my youth. It worked so well that people started arriving just to watch, but soon found themselves borrowing spoons and forks from anyone with extras just so they could try it themselves.

Children were particularly good, not yet understanding that this kind of thing is impossible. Soon Jack was forced to raid flea markets in his off-hours, acquiring boxes of old silverware and kitchen utensils for those who showed up empty handed.

Needless to say, hardly anyone left those evenings without a pretzel-shaped kitchen utensil or six in their pockets – I've still got mine after all these years – plus the new-found knowledge that it doesn't take a Uri Gellar to bend a spoon bowl in half with your mind. I've seen children eight years old bend half-inch diameter rods, and once watched a frail grandmother in her eighties curl up a salad fork in half a minute flat. Once it starts, it's gone!

Over the years Jack's been doing this I'm sure he's acquired 90% of the discarded silverware in the Southern California area, as he's conducted evening after evening teaching people that the limits of their minds aren't limits at all, but just milestones.

Jack took the same approach to firewalking. Having visited several firewalks among native cultures around the world, his scientist's mind went to work, not to duplicate the feat himself, but rather wondering what the actual temperature of the walker's foot sole was during the walk.

He designed and built special thermistors that measure temperature and then transmit it to a read-out some (cooler) distance away, then he attached them to the feet of the firewalkers. He soon discovered that while the fiery red coals themselves were more than 400 (Fahrenheit) degrees hot, the soles of the feet that touched them remained around 100°F!

So astrophysicist Jack Houck is an interesting man, to say the least, and on that stressful night in 1984, knowing that he did interesting – some would say impossible – things, I wanted to talk to him about my eye. I cornered him at the Schwartz's party over a glass of wine, and told him my tale of woe, that two of the best eye specialists in the country had told me I was going to lose the vision in my right eye.

His response took all of ten seconds. He just looked at me and laughed. Then, like the preachers of my youth, he put his hand on my forehead, but he didn't invoke any power from on high, nor did me slap me to the ground with the force of the divine. He simply said, "Ben, you know better than that. Don't you remember? Your eye is fine. You just forgot, didn't you?"

In that moment a rush of emotion swept over me just like I used to see happen in the revival tents. I was "touched" from my head to my toes, and I broke down in tears. Somehow, right there, something deep inside me realized that I had in fact just forgotten that my eye was really perfect.

I had listened to others, rather than understanding the truth. "Yes, I understand. Thank you," I said, and hugged him gratefully. It was as if my tears were washing away the problem in my eye. But more than that. They were freeing me from fear and allowing my body to heal itself, completely unimpeded by, or maybe aided by, my mind.

I felt I had been in the hands of a healer, and I said so. Jack laughed again, and said, "No, it's not me, it's you, Ben. You didn't need me for anything more than to remind you of what you already knew."

By the next morning, the spider web was gone, and it never came back. A year later I went for a regular eye exam and my vision was 20-20. Twenty years after that evening the vision in my right eye – in both eyes – is 20-30, according to my most recent aviator's flight physical. And there's no such thing as a macular pucker in either eye.

I never went back to the specialist who had asked me to return after six months if I could still see. I didn't need to prove anything to him, and I didn't want to be near any place where I had experienced a lack of surety that my eye was perfect.

As the great Dr. Albert Schweitzer said, "Each patient carries his own doctor inside him."

If we can only access it.

◊

Casual Magic

One summer during college, I was a cameraman for a television station in Jacksonville, Florida. One day I was working on one of the talk shows we aired live in our studio, when a fascinating guest was brought on: a man who could chew up light bulbs.

These were the days when fluoroscopes were still in vogue – the green 3' x 3' X-ray machine which, when you stepped into it, painted an image of your insides on the screen in front of you. It was banned years ago, along with the popular X-ray device used in shoe stores which showed you your foot – and your foot bones – inside a shoe. It was pretty cool, though. (Sometimes science takes one step forward and marketing makes it two steps back.)

On this day, Mr. Smith, we'll call him (I've long since forgotten his name), proudly demonstrated his strange ability to all of us in the studio and to the Jacksonville television audience, to crunch up glass and metal with his teeth and swallow them right down. The show's host took out a couple sixty watt GE light bulbs recently purchased at the local grocery, and Mr. Smith proceeded to bite into them, glass first, and chew them up. The metal bases took a little extra crunching, but he got them down, too, and then the host examined him.

I was the fortunate camera to take the close-up of his mouth – no blood, no torn tissue, just a few small pieces of glass he quickly finished up. Live on TV, mind you! Then he stepped into the fluoroscope, and Camera 2 got a full-screen shot of the man's central organs, *focusing on his stomach, where clear evidence of the crunched-up metal bases lay. The other two cameramen, me being one, plus the stage manager, the lighting director, the producer and half a dozen station employees all stepped up to the fluoroscope to get a better look. We were all amazed.*

After the show was over, several of us crowded around Mr. Smith, asking him to "do it again," and he obliged. This time I got a full-frontal look as he bit into a perfectly good light bulb, chewed it up and swallowed it, picking a few shards of glass out of his teeth with his fingernail for dessert, just as before, no blood, no torn tissue, and no sign of distress.

Then, as a capper, he continued to chat with us about how he had come to this strange calling as he took out a 12-inch long knitting needle and in one smooth move jammed it completely through his left arm. All of us reeled back in shock, and a couple of people nearly lost their lunch. Once again, no bleeding and no apparent pain, and I was two feet away. When he pulled it out, there was barely a mark where it had been.

We asked him how he did this, and he smiled and said, "Well, I pick up the knitting needle like this and jab it into my arm like this," doing it again. I think my own arm went numb with pain about then.

Then he told us he didn't know how it was that he could do either of those things. He'd been able to do them for as long as he could remember, and as he grew older he himself wondered how he could do it when no one else could. He had come to realize that there was some kind of automatic preparation, a "knowingness" that it was not going to hurt him, but he didn't know where it came from. Something in him said "this is going to be fun," each time, and it was.

A few years later I saw someone else, on NBC's Saturday Night Live, do the needle through the arm demonstration—horrifying the first five rows of the audience, by the way – but I've never since see anyone eat light bulbs since that day in Jacksonville.

Chapter II: Conversations with a Mole

During that period in my life when I was competitively single and concerned more about my body than my mind, a mole suddenly erupted on my forehead. It was only a little knot of a thing, emerging from under the skin, but it was "right where everyone could see it!" and I didn't like it. Every time I looked in the mirror it frustrated me. At first I thought of having it cut off, but I figured there would always be a little scar, and I didn't want a scar, either.

I decided it was time to take some serious action. Just as the lazy man makes the best inventor, I guess there's nothing like a minor physical imperfection to drive a vain man to innovation.

It wasn't long after my amazing experience with my eye. The magic of that healing had emboldened me along the path of "I am my own healer," so using the techniques I had learned from a few meditation classes, modified with my own years of irrational, poorly educated and probably misguided thinking on the subject, I sat down on the floor in a quiet room, took myself into as deep a meditative state as I knew how, and began to roam my mind around my body. You probably know the drill, "Imagine your feet relaxed…imagine your ankles relaxed, imagine your legs relaxed, imagine the two big lumps on your rear relaxed, etc."

I was in too much a hurry for all this, so I just soared up my face, to that vicious little blob of a sphere on my skin, and sat down beside it, thinking I was going to "imagine it gone." But this time I did something different:

Without thinking much about it, I said out loud, "What are you doing here?" I didn't expect a response, I was just frustrated.

"You invited me," was the surprising answer. It didn't come in words, exactly, it was more like the idea just popped into my head.

"Really? Why?" I responded, again out loud. Lucky I was somewhere where no one could hear me. I've always worried the Mental

Normalcy Patrol would some day find me and haul me off to the Institution for the Idiotically Insane (appropriately, the "I-I-I").

"Only you know that," it answered.

"Oh, thanks. Well, you can leave now, or I'm going to have you cut out."

"That's not necessary."

"Oh, I know it's not necessary, but I don't want you on my face."

"Where do you want me? On your butt? Some inoperable location in your body?"

"Why are you doing this?"

"Because you invited me here…you asked me to come for some reason, and I came."

"Why?"

"I don't know that, I'm just a blob on your forehead. You're the brains around here."

"Well I changed my mind. You can leave now."

The blob shrugged.

That was about it for session one. I zoomed up out of my meditation and washed my face, trying to imagine I didn't do what I just did. I had an otherwise commonplace day at work, but unfortunately every so often I had to go to the bathroom, and I couldn't help stealing a glimpse in the mirror as I washed my hands. Had it actually talked to me? Had I actually invited it to appear on my face? To teach me something! What a concept.

A week later the blob was bigger than ever. Not terribly big, mind you, but too big. I was sure now that everywhere I went people were surreptitiously glancing at it, and laughing or feeling sorry for me behind my back. Did I mention I was vain?

After a couple weeks of living with it, I figured, what's the worse that can happen if I get in there and try to make friends with it and fail?

I can always revert to my previous universe and go have it taken off. And in that universe I don't believe that a little innocuous mole on my forehead portends metastasized cancer and painful death anyway – do I? I believe it's just a mole, and if I get it looked at (quickly!!) it can be dealt with and that's that.

Well, I will admit that there was a possibility of the terror inside me (of a painful death from cancer that I could have caught in time but decided to do such a stupid thing as talking to it instead, while it grew large, ugly tentacles into my brain and sucked the life out of me)…yes, of that terror welling up and clouding my brain and overcoming my entire life…BUT, instead of doing that, when no one else was home, I went into my bedroom, sat down on the floor, closed my eyes, hurried into meditation – bypassing yet again the "imagine your spleen relaxed" part – made myself small and zoomed up next to my Mole and sat down again.

"You still here?" I said.

It shrugged (I imagined). After a long moment I added, "I thought maybe we could be friends."

"Friends, now. Why?"

"Because you're hanging around my body and I figured we might as well get acquainted…we're pretty intimate already, under the circumstances."

"Well you're afraid of me."

"I know. I guess that's stupid, huh?"

"Yep."

There's a start! I admitted to my mole I was afraid of it! Scary.

I asked it again what it was doing here, and it only replied that I had to figure it out for myself. It suddenly seemed like one of those children's fairy tales, "If you can't guess why I'm here in three tries, I'm going to destroy your face."

So I sat there on the floor of my bedroom, eyes closed, imagination perched somewhere on the front of my forehead beside my mole. I looked at it, growing out of perfectly normal undertissue. I got closer, noticed the cells. They looked fine to me. "You guys okay?" I asked. "Yeah, sure. As if you ever cared until now," came the imagined answer.

"What are you doing here, then?" Here we go again.

"We're not here, it's just your imagination." Well that was different, at least.

"So if I have imagined you here, why can't I imagine you gone?"

"What will take our place?"

"Normal skin."

"We are normal. Perfect, in fact."

Hmmm. That made me stop a moment. There was something in one of the books I'd read, or lectures I'd been to with some woman I was trying to impress…if I could only remember…something like, if God is perfect, and I am already a perfect manifestation of God in the physical, therefore all this stuff I think of as good and bad has to already be perfect in some fundamental, metaphysical sense. So my mole is perfect and…*what the hell is all this perfection anyway, who needs it, we know life's not perfect, for God's sake, this is all so new age-y boring and I just want to go have this thing cut out and be done with it!!!*

Okay, okay, okay. I've vented. Back to the dialogue with my mole:

"So why do I want a mole on my face." Pause. Contemplation. Then…a hint:

"What would you be doing now if I weren't here?"

"Probably chasing women or out trying to make a buck..."

"Right."

"Right what?"

"Right, so…do I have to make it as clear as the mole on your face for you?"

"So I wouldn't be sitting here on the floor talking to myself, is that what you're saying?"

Now it suddenly turned shrink on me: "Is that what you're saying?"

"Shut up. I'm the only one talking, I guess so." But the thought made me laugh. "Okay, so you're here to get my attention so I will sit down on the floor and talk to you and think of these things I'm thinking of, is that it?"

"Everything you have ever done has led you to this moment." The Philosopher Mole!

"Okay, so will you go away, then?"

"Make me."

I sat there frustrated for a moment, then remembered my own new age-y sweetness and light find-the-good-in-everyone philosophy, which I thought was probably a good way to live and promised I'd try to practice someday. I said aloud, "Gosh, Mole, thank you for being here, I really appreciate you coming to make me stop and think about these things. Now you can return to God, or subsume into the rest of the cells of the body."

I didn't believe it, of course. I knew the blob wasn't going anywhere, it was just going to get bigger everyday until it took over my face and I became Elephant Man and people shielded their eyes from me when I passed or I died a horribly gruesome death during which no one would come to visit me in the hospital – and this was because I had led such a vain, selfish life, never doing anything for anyone but myself. Did I mention I was a hypochondriac (and melodramatic)? As I'm sure you know by now, it comes from my mother's side of the family.

I sat for a while longer, and tried again. "I really mean it. Thank you for the lesson. You can go now, I have learned it. I understand." And I said it again. And strangely, the more I said it, the more I actually came to mean it. And as I meant it more and more, I also realized for the first time that it was possible the mole would disappear.

It was six weeks before it was completely gone. Each day I would look in the mirror and thank it for having come to teach me that I could talk to it, and remind it that it was now okay to go.

It finally completely vanished. When it was gone, I kept checking for weeks after, a part of me still astonished that this had happened. A year later, there was not even the tiniest sign on my forehead that anything like that ever grew there. Even these many years later, you might catch me looking to make sure every once in awhile, if you're quick.

What really happened? Everyone will have a different opinion, because we all live in different universes, where such a thing is either possible, or not. Some will think it was a miracle. Some will believe this could have happened if I had seen a healer, or an evangelist, or been to Lourdes. Some will believe it would have gone away anyway, naturally, whether I talked to it or not. And some will believe I made up this story, for they will not be able to conceive a world in which something like this could happen.

But it did.

Our concept of reality is really based on the bombastic input of our five powerful senses, plus the fact that our conscious minds are not very good at multidimensional conceptualizing. That is, we are overloaded with sensory input and can really only focus on one thing at a time. So anything else going on takes a back seat.

We tend to suppress the quiet subtleties around us – in fact most of us ignore them altogether. So if you're in a cocktail party filled with rock music, fifty people talking and the energy of social intercourse, you're probably not going to notice your stomach growling, much less your liver quietly getting anxious over that third drink you just inhaled.

I liken it to standing near a runway at an airport and trying to hold a conversation. So long as no big jets are taking off, you can carry on a dialogue quite easily. But let one of those noisy giants power up and start its takeoff roll, and quickly the tones of your casual conversation are impossible to hear. They're still in there, but buried now by the overpowering stimulus of the jet roar.

We are not capable of sensing small details when a large detail takes up all our sensory capability. In today's world, we seem to live in sensory overload most of the time. So I guess we're not going to notice it if a stupid mole on our face wants to talk to us.

For millennia our sages have told us to "be still and know," find that quiet place and close the door and pray, or meditate, or take a vacation. Interesting things can be heard when we do.

If we believe the postulates of quantum theory, and the writings of countless mystics and wise people, some part of us understands that what we experience as physical reality is not necessarily really physical – nor real – at all. That we are truly made up of "nothing, in particular." But the "in particular" is important. It's the particular stuff of "us," somehow differentiating us from "not us." So if I'm not really real – physical – then that mole on my forehead isn't real, either. Not, at least, in the sense where I need to worry about it being permanent.

And if it and I aren't really real, then why can't I talk to it – anthropomorphize it, so to speak? I mean we talk to our pets, don't we? And for at least several thousand years we have anthropomorphized our deities. If a mole on the forehead of a human isn't human, what is it?

Oh, I know, it doesn't have a brain to think with, nor a mouth to talk with, etc. But maybe it does: it's connected pretty intimately to my own brain and mouth. So where does the mole stop and I begin?

"I and my mole are one." Or, "my mole speaks through me." I must admit it certainly affected my speech, and my thoughts, for sure. The difference between having it and not having it was precisely what I thought other people were thinking because I had it. So it clearly communicated with me! Okay, you say, "No, it didn't communicate with you, you reacted to it." I say, what's the practical difference?

And since science and religion taught me that my consciousness isn't bound by the limitations of physical size and shape, or even time, why can't I shuttle on up to my forehead and sit down next to this mole and find out what's up?

If we consider the possibility that everything that happens to us is caused maybe just in part by our actions, reactions and thoughts – plus mix in a bit of "why God brought me here" and what the heck, reincarnation, maybe, if you're into karma – then maybe there is a reason this mole sneaked up there and planted itself on my forehead – and maybe I'm just too stupid to consider that this might be the way the Maker really works.

Maybe it goes like this: "Okay, I'll give you a small nudge, and if you don't get that, I'll give you a bigger one, and if that doesn't work, here comes the Big C."

The question was, of course, "Get What?" So then, I'm really nervous. "OMG, if I don't figure this mole thing out, something really terrible is going to happen." I felt like a novice jumping out of an airplane without having been taught how to open the parachute.

But, isn't that exactly how life feels? Like we were dumped here and they forgot to send down the instructions for how to work everything out? And maybe the Bible or the Koran or the Bhagavad Gita has them but we're not sure whose interpretation to believe so ultimately we have to figure it out ourselves, and most of the people who say they have figured it out don't know shit...? So we all get nervous and terrified and greedy and we stake out our territory and then realize we have to work together to get anything done but we don't trust "them" and they don't trust us so we become devious and gang up while still trying to be friends because underneath it all we really know that Love is the way but we're afraid to let down our guard and see what would happen because it might kill us.

Kinda like the "Survivor" TV show, isn't it? So terrified we're going to be kicked off this beautiful island called earth that we dare not take time to explore all of life's amazing possibilities...

...like talking to a mole.

For years after the success with the mole, now armed with two successful magical experiences, I privately practiced this technique with practically every fear and health issue I faced. While runners took a week off when their knees started to give them pain, I ran and "talked my knee out of it." When I'd cut myself slicing an apple in the kitchen, I'd wash the wound, close it carefully with my fingers, then imagine going inside, to the cells around the cut, and talk to them, soothing them from their shock before putting on a bandage.

As I became more practiced, and more comfortable that this worked, sometimes I wouldn't need a bandage on a small cut, it would close quickly enough on its own – certainly not like that guy in Jacksonville who could chew up light bulbs without drawing blood, but kind of in that direction...a little. I mean, if he could do it *big time*, then maybe I could do it *little time*.

A banged shin would get special attention from me for a minute or so, rubbed from the outside and caressed from the inside, and it would recover quickly.

It's as if I was getting my fear out of the way so the body could do what it knows to do – or in reverse, when I allowed my fear to influence what should have been a simple matter, I was getting in the way, and slowing the healing down.

Over the years I learned to talk most headaches away with only a minute or two of attention, and I spent years during my daily run talking to every part of my body. I ran near a noisy freeway, and I'd wait until I was far away from anyone who could hear me, and then I'd start talking. <u>Out loud</u>.

You can, too.

◊

Casual Magic

A few years ago I learned about a Russian healer who had just arrived in Los Angeles and was gathering fame as not only being a good healer, but he supposedly could move objects on a table by just putting his hand close to them. Being still the curious skeptic, but allowing all things to be possible in the Universe, I called him up, introduced myself as a documentary filmmaker interested in doing a film on him, and asked him to lunch. We met at Jerry's Deli in Studio City, one of the busiest and most public places in the city.

He was a young man, probably no older than 30, tall, with a mischievous smile. We talked over sandwiches and egg creams about his "gift." He told me he grew up in Russia, during the Soviet Union era; his family lived in the country outside of Moscow. He said he was a normal kid until shortly after his ninth birthday. One night while he was asleep, for apparently no particular reason, a bright light came in through his bedroom window and woke him. He said the light "filled the room," and he felt it fill him, as well. He said it "told" him that he was going to be a healer, and then it left and he fell back to sleep. When he woke up he discovered had these strange and wonderful abilities.

And then he proceeded to demonstrate one of them to me. For starters, he held up his right hand and said, "Examine my hand, do you see anything unusual about it?" Of course I did not, it looked like *an ordinary man's hand. He turned it over, opened his fingers, and showed me that it was empty. And he was wearing a short-sleeved shirt; nothing up his sleeves either. Then he reached across the table and put his hand about an inch above the restaurant's bottle of Heinz Ketchup, and I watched in amazement as the glass bottle rose to meet his hand and attach itself at the cap to his open palm, as if a magnet were pulling it upwards. Holding his palm flat and parallel with the table, the bottle still firmly attached, he raised the bottle higher above the table and moved it to me. "Take it," he said. I reached out, grasped the bottle and tried to take it, but I couldn't pull it away from his hand. He relaxed his hand slightly and said, "Now," and the bottle fell into my hand. Then he turned his palm to me, to show me again that there was nothing in it.*

"Give me that hand," I said. He laughed and held both hands out to me; he'd been challenged many times before. I looked at them, felt them, and concluded once again that they were normal human hands. He shrugged, "I bond with the object. In my mind, I experience a connection with it, and it comes to me. I don't know how I do it."

"Give me your pen," he said. I took my ordinary ball point pen out of my pocket and handed it to him. He took it, stretched out his hand again, palm down, and placed the pen underneath the outstretched palm, horizontally. And it stayed there. Then, from about six inches away, he waved the fingers of his left hand, as if instructing the pen to move, and it moved, rolling underneath his arm all the way to the elbow. My pen.

"Now you do it," he instructed me. I laughed. "No, seriously. Stretch out your hand like mine." I did so, stretching it out over the table. "Take the pen," he said, "and do what I did." So I took the pen, and placed it underneath my outstretched palm, and let go. It fell to the table. He laughed. "Try it again."

This time he put his hand on top of mine. I put the pen underneath my palm again, and now it stayed! My hand didn't feel any different than before, but with his hand on top of mine, the pen was staying against my palm just like he had done.

"Now you keep it," he ordered. And he removed his hand from mine.

And for the next 30 seconds or so, that common writing pen I had taken out of my pocket stayed attached under my open palm no matter how I moved. Then it gradually became less sticky, and nothing I could do could kept it attached. It fell off, onto the table. I picked it up and tried it again myself, and it wouldn't stay.

I've never been able to do it again.

Chapter III: Altering States

Until the television set became a fixture in most people's homes, travelers would return from trips to strange and distant lands with stories of people who could do marvelous, almost unimaginable things. At will they could lower their blood pressure, their heart rate and their breathing to near death-like levels. They could be buried alive and survive. Documentary films were made showing someone preparing himself, then being put into a box no bigger than his body, and buried alive. When hours or days later the box was dug up and opened, the man would emerge from the experience apparently no worse for the wear.

These were astonishing examples of what we are capable of, but no one I knew considered them more than mere carnival side shows. And in an unlucky trick of language, the men who performed these feats were known as *fakirs*, which in Arabic merely means *poor man*.[10] I suspect the name was too close to the English word "faker" to avoid a permanent negative connotation. Down deep our mid-20th century culture couldn't really accept that this kind of thing was even possible.

In the Pentecostal church of the mid-20th century, long before Western medicine had any handle on cancer, heart disease, or the common cold for that matter, faith healing was rather routine. The novel and movie "Elmer Gantry" and, later, Robert Duvall's "The Apostle," portrayed it vividly. We have all seen the classic version: a tent meeting where a sweaty, high-voltage evangelist in crisp white shirt, rolled up sleeves, collar open, tie askew, grabs the head of a suffering saint and rocks him back and forth while invoking JE-sus! and HE-yal! and lets him collapse in a heap on the revival floor, only to have the healee jump up shouting and running around the tent declaring "I'm healed, thank you Jesus I'm healed!"

---

[10] In Hindu it is *religious mendicant (beggar) wonder worker*.

It happened frequently, and not only in tent meetings like that one. So many occurrences of it were documented over the years that medicine coined a phrase for it: *instantaneous remission*. Cancer and tumors seemed to be the main serious diseases made to disappear, but arthritis, gout, bum legs, bad backs and other maladies were frequently cured, too. Faith healing worked then and it does today, producing frequent short-term healings and the occasional permanent healing – and no one ever seems to know which, if anything, is going to be the result when.

Recently an astounding item appeared in the news: *"Oscar Winners Live Longer!"* A study of several hundred Academy Award winners over the years indicated that they tend to live an average of 3.9 years longer than non-winners – six years if they win more than one! Something about the inner peace and self-esteem that winning the golden statue gives them?

I'll vouch for that. Once a documentary film I had made was a finalist at the Emmy Awards in Hollywood. Throughout the dinner and speeches that preceded the naming of the recipient of the award (the Television Academy doesn't like to say "winner," but I will), I sat at my table sneezing and coughing, nursing a full-blown case of the flu combined with the worst cold I'd had in years. By the time they got around to announcing the winner, I had gone through a full box of tissues and was surreptitiously eyeing the edge of the tablecloth lying in my lap. And then: "The Emmy goes to…(more sneezing and blowing of the nose)…Ben Moses!"

Shocked, I rose from the table, made my way to the podium, accepted the award, gave a small terrified speech, and returned to my table filled with astonishment and glee. My wife congratulated me and held out a new tissue. And at that moment I realized that my nose was clear, my chest was clear, my head no longer hurt…I felt GREAT! *Healed*, even.

I basked in the healthy glow of winning that award the rest of the year. It was a long time before I got sick again.

The Other 90% of the Brain

The famous maxim, attributed to Albert Einstein, that we are only using 10% of the capacity of our brain, is oft quoted and seldom acted upon. Not that we don't want to, we just don't know how. But in the mid 1940's, José Silva, a Laredo, Texas electronics technician, was watching his young children struggle with their homework and wanted to find a way to help them learn better.

Silva had studied extensively in the fields of psychology and parapsychology, and decided to apply his knowledge to try and help the children assimilate information more efficiently. The right-brain intuitive techniques he developed worked so well that soon he was asked to help other kids, and he gradually began teaching the process to others. In the early '60s he offered the method to the government, but was politely rejected. Nevertheless, the demand for his classes had become so great that he recruited teachers and formalized his learning system as The Silva Method, eventually offering it worldwide.

He called his process of applying the mind "Mind Control," an unfortunate choice of labels in that period between the Korean War and Vietnam, when accusations were flowing out of Asia of Chinese soldiers using 'brainwashing' techniques – often called "mind control." This fact, plus a general suspicion of the hypnosis techniques used in the program,[11] gave Silva's course title a not-so-pleasant ring. Many people were turned off by it.

But the process itself was profound. His technique proposed a new way of looking at the world. He invited students to temporarily set aside their preconceived ideas of how reality worked, and "play" in a new imaginary paradigm for awhile. His teachers added, "You can always go back to your old reality when you leave."

The course was promoted as something to help you expand the possibilities in your life; to help you learn and work better. But

---

[11] Hypnosis had already been tried in psychotherapy with inconsistent results.

the process was far more interesting than its advertising suggested. The games you were invited to play in this invented reality included imagining that you could shrink yourself to be as small as the inside of a leaf, or peer inside your pet's body to see how it worked or even to see if something was wrong.

During the course, students spent hours with their eyes closed, working to the tick of a metronome in a deep "theta" level of relaxation, constructing in their minds a very detailed "room," outfitted with every conceivable imaginary device for instantly traveling through space and time, and for making themselves larger or smaller, at will, in order to observe the unobservable: the space and sounds within a rock, the feelings within a mind, the artery walls surrounding a heart.

In their mental room, Silva's students imagined they could look at anyone or anything they chose, from far or near, past or present. In this new universe they had made up, they could notice areas of injury or disease, or they could "put on someone's head" (why not?) to get a feeling of who they were, how they looked at life, how tense or relaxed they were, and even what muscle tone was different than their own. One student, given the name of another's friend as a test subject, playfully "put on" the subject's head and immediately recognized this person as a guitarist – because his own arm and hand muscles involuntarily tensed and curled as if holding a guitar.

Given only the name and date of birth, another student imagined the female subject to have a swollen, heavy left arm, one breast missing – "cut out," he said – and a terribly unhappy outlook on life. He "saw" that she was dressed in a long, black and white outfit, with white "wings" for a hat. Upon debriefing, he was informed that the woman in question was a nun and had recently undergone a radical mastectomy of the left breast. The heavy arm was due to edema from the operation. The depressed attitude the student perceived needed no explanation.

Another student was asked to describe a friend's brother, and when the student "put on" the brother's head he found himself somehow unable to speak until he made the physical gesture of "taking off the head." The friend then told him that his brother was presently in the hospital, in catatonic shock. He had overdosed on drugs the night before.

A Silva student was given the name and date of birth of an eight-year old boy by the class instructor. The observer closed his eyes, descended into his "room," and sought out the child. The first image that came to mind was the boy running after a baseball as it jumped a curb and rolled into the street. He saw the boy run headlong into the street after it, then he saw the shiny bumper of a car, and suddenly a deep indentation in the boy's skull. Not understanding anything more than this image in his mind's eye, the student remarked, "That's too hard a hit, you can't survive a hit like that." The instructor said, "All, right, so what do you see?" The student shook his head, "His forehead is pushed in from the bumper. He has to be dead."

The instructor acknowledged that this was so. "It happened this year," he said, "can you tell me the month?" The student didn't know how to find that information. "Just look at his life energy month to month, starting in January, and see what happens."

The student, eyes still tightly closed, imagined seeing the boy in January of that year and sensed a strong energy about him as if he was running and playing. He moved his imagination to February and still felt the intense energy of the child. March, April, May…all vibrant, alive. And then June…and the energy stopped cold, as if beautiful music had suddenly stopped playing. All was quiet. "He died in June," he said.

It was so. The instructor told him that in early June of that year that little boy had been hit by a car as he chased a ball into the street, and had died.

The instructor was the boy's uncle. The student who was seeing – imagining – all of those things, the nun, the catatonic brother, the boy hit by the car, was...*me*.

Nowhere in my life had I been prepared for the possibility that we could do such things; that our imagination, so directed, could point us to reality. But after that "Silva Mind Control Course," I was forced to admit possibilities I had never conceived of before. I had to alter my perception of reality yet again.

That profound experience led to many more sessions like that over the years, experiments in proving to myself, a man rooted in classic Bible Belt tradition, that all of this actually was possible...and verifiable. Long after the course was over, I worked with some of my Silva classmates as we continually demonstrated to ourselves that we, ordinary people, were actually doing verifiable "psychic readings" as we called them.

Not too many years later, the kind of experimenting we were doing underwent serious scientific study, helped in great part by the work of Ingo Swan[12] and later Stephan Schwartz and others, plus the revelation that the U.S. government was studying it, as well, at SRI, the Stanford Research Institute. Swan dubbed it "remote viewing," and today it is widely accepted as a natural ability of the mind, usually undeveloped by most of us. As with any other of our natural talents, like singing, for example, some people are better at it than others, but all of us can at least "carry a tune" in the remote viewing realm, if we only set our minds to it.

Stephan Schwartz proved this on national television several times. I participated in one demonstration in the '80s, when at the request of Westinghouse's Group W Broadcasting, Stephan set up a remove viewing experiment for the television cameras. Under strict observance by Group W executives and direct control of

---

[12] Ingo Swan was a Swedish delegate to the United Nations who, in the early 1970s, proved to have an uncanny ability at "remote viewing" and set out protocols for conducting experiments. He took his work to SRI, and thus began a scientific probe into this "sixth sense."

Harry Blackstone, Jr., a well-known magician and unyielding skeptic, Blackstone locked Stephan and several of us test subjects in a room, including a Group W vice president who had never heard of this stuff before. Also locked in with us was a Group W camera crew, recording everything. Blackstone stayed outside the room.

Once we were secured, Blackstone instructed a second camera crew to get in their van and drive away. Somewhere on the road they should decide on a public place to go. A few minutes later they called Blackstone, telling him they were at the destination. b*ut not telling him where they were.*

Blackstone called through the locked door to Stephan that we should begin. Stephan handed us all blank sheets of paper and told us to draw a picture of our imaginings of where the television crew was at that moment. "You have ten minutes," he said. As we drew our scenes on paper, the TV crew with us filmed. At the end of the time, each of us signed our names to our drawings, Stephan collected the papers and we waited. Five minutes later, by predetermined schedule, the remote TV crew called Blackstone again and announced their location. Then the door was unlocked, Stephan handed our drawings to Blackstone, and everyone, including the TV crew in the room, followed the renowned skeptic to the location the traveling crew had picked: the Los Angeles Zoo.

Standing at the zoo's entrance, the show's host and Blackstone held up the drawings we had made. The correlation of randomly drawn pictures and the actual location was uncanny, so accurate that even avowed skeptic Blackstone could easily see that we all had drawn various aspects of the LA Zoo.

Needless to say, the Group W vice president was the most surprised of all, because his drawing, too, was clearly of the zoo, and until that moment he had had no idea of any ability to do such a thing. Blackstone admitted on camera that he had never witnessed such a thing before either, and he was sure there had been no way for us to know of the location before or during the experiment. He didn't know how it was done, but he knew there had been no cheating.

Until Schwartz started conducting these demonstrations on television, and the government admitted it was doing them, too, remote viewing was considered pretty spooky, even by those of us involved. We didn't talk about it to too many people.

In New York, in the latter part of our Silva training, we were told to bring to class a few 3x5 inch file cards on which we had written people's names, dates of birth, and pertinent personal or health information about them. We were to only use people no one else in the group could possibly know. That was easy for me, I was fresh from my hometown in the Midwest; no one would know any of my friends from there. As further test of this strange ability all of us were learning how to use, at least one of the names was to be of someone who was no longer alive.

I remember one particularly powerful session, in which I gave my assigned partner the name and date of birth of a man about my own age, someone I had known since I was six. Sitting on the floor, she closed her eyes and drifted into her mental room to seek out this stranger and tell me about him. She began in the way we were taught, describing his features as best she could, but it was her description of him as a teenager playing with horses in a field filled with "blue grass" that captured my attention. It took me a moment before I remembered that when he was 15, his family had moved to Kentucky – the "Bluegrass State" – where they had bought a farm.

I asked her to move forward in time, to see him present day. We had gone to grade school together, he would have been 30 or so, now. She was quiet for awhile, and then said she couldn't find him. I asked her to go back in time until she could find him, and tell me what he was doing and how old he was.

Once again she sat quietly for a period, and then said, "There he is…he's about 21. I see him running across a grassy field…over a small hill. He's wearing light tan shirt and pants, and carrying something…ohh, he's falling into the grass…it's strange…now there's a hole in his chest…"

When he was 22, my childhood best friend Bill Settlemire was killed in Vietnam.

◊

> "... *quantum mechanics does not represent particles, but rather, our knowledge, our observations, or our <u>consciousness</u> of particles.*"
>
> - Werner Heisenberg, "The Representation of Nature in Contemporary Physics," *Daedalus*, 87:3, (Summer, 1958), pp. 95-108. © 1958 by the American Academy of Arts & Sciences.

Chapter IV: The Other Half of Reality

I must admit I had trouble accepting the idea that anyone besides Edgar Cayce or certain special people like him could do psychic readings, remote viewing, or whatever you want to call this "magic." And over the years since I first learned how to do it, I have shied away from any public acknowledgement of this ability, all the while preaching to anyone who would listen that everyone has this potential.

But at the same time, I was completely accepting of another form of magic – and found it not the slightest bit strange that it worked for me, as it does for everyone. I was first licensed as an amateur radio operator – a "Ham" – at age 10 when, as a Boy Scout, I became fascinated with the fact that invisible radio waves deliver words and music – and pictures even – across hundreds and thousands of miles. Certainly in the 1800s, the time of Guglielmo Marconi[13], the concept of radio waves traveling through the air was nearly impossible to accept; it was scoffed at and denied, just as magic as the idea that "mental waves" (or whatever they are) might do the same thing.

What's even more impossible to grasp, these magical radio waves are created with rocks, sand and metal.

In their simplest form, the electronic communication methods we take for granted work because there exists in the ground a particular kind of common rock – a mica crystal – which, when a tiny electromagnetic force is impressed upon it, will start to vibrate and, depending on the size of the crystal, will vibrate a specific number of times per second for as long as the force is on it. Not only does the crystal vibrate, but somehow so do the electrons in the long thin piece of copper wire which is attached to it (copper from the ground, of course), and that wire can be connected to

---

[13] Italian pioneer in long-distance radio transmission (1874-1937).

another particular piece of rock, which is glued to some compressed sand (we call it silicon), which in turn is glued to the first kind of rock, and when different electromagnetic forces are put on one side or another of the rocks, the vibration carried by the electrons which were stimulated by the force which passed through the crystal can be magnified to such a large extent that when you connect another copper wire to one of the other rocks, by way of a couple other thin pieces of copper that aren't even connected to each other but only wound close to each other (!), and then hang the second long piece of wire out of a window, the tiny crystal's magnified vibrations somehow go up to the sky and some 50 miles up they somehow bounce off of minute parts of atoms (ions) floating up there, and careen back to earth thousands of miles away, and they do all this at the speed of light!

Impossible? No. *Ordinary* magic. As compared to *extraordinary* magic, which is different, of course, because we haven't accepted it yet.

Everything around us is filled with radio waves, delivering information, music, conversations, pictures, from TV and radio transmitters, conversations with space stations, telephone links from microwave dishes, radar signals from our semi- and self-driving cars, chats and selfies from our smart phones, from one point to another, often thousands of miles away – and millions of miles out into space. And, of course, at the other end – or at this end, or almost anywhere, for that matter, more rocks and sand and metal can be shaped and formed and connected in such a way that those incredibly fainter-than-faint vibrations bouncing off of the ions in the sky are transformed into vibrations on a piece of plastic or paper (a "speaker" or headphones) so that someone sitting near it can actually hear and make sense of them just as they were spoken into the magic machine thousands of miles away a nanosecond earlier!

Magic. The universe is so filled with magic and mysteries that no matter how much we think we know about it, it remains fundamentally unknowable. We learn more every day, but with each bit of additional knowledge comes the realization that it is more vast and mysteriously complex than we ever thought.

Last month, the earth was flat and the sky a firmament with holes filled with light. The sun traveled across the sky in a chariot, and Queen Nut ruled the darkness.

Last week, the sky was made up of fiery hot stars surrounded by vast empty space, and the solar system was the only place in the universe that had planets.

Yesterday those stars got neighbors: pulsars, quasars, supernovas and dark stars, and they mostly all have planets, and the empty space is filled with black holes, dark matter and anti-matter particles, a strong force, a weak force, and solar wind.

And today? Today we may discover that this dance we do with our bodies is a **pas de deux** *between consciousness and energy which is eminently alterable by the power of our words.*

A dance? An amazingly intricate dance. Consider that the earth is turning on its north-south axis at 600+ miles per hour. We are not standing motionless on the earth, we are whirling at close to the speed of sound on the outside of a 24,000-mile-around sphere. Worse yet, this spinning earth is spiraling around the sun at 66,630 miles per hour. But wait, there's more. The sun and all of its children are moving in yet another huge circle around the center of the Milky Way, at 3,600,000 miles per hour! That's ten thousand miles per second, if you care.

So now you know that when you tuck your kids in at night, you're a liar if you tell them, "I'll be right here, I'm not going anyplace, don't you worry."

Oops, we didn't add the fact that our Milky Way galaxy is moving around the center of the known universe at some god-awful speed…

Hold on, we're not done...According to the Big Bang theory, everything is moving away from itself an astronomical number of megamiles per second. Gotta factor that in!

Okay. So at any given moment, although we may think we're perfectly still, our bodies are going forward, or backward, or flipping up, or down, or around, one way then the next – always in motion. And that's just the outside. No wonder we're always so confused. Vertigo, anyone?

Most people believe that because of the overwhelming force of earth's gravity, we don't feel these smaller movements, and they have no particular influence on our lives. But science describes something called centripetal force, which is an outward pressure exerted on a mass when it is whirled around a central point. I would venture that in the case of all these various spins happening to us, the resultant pressures are something we feel but suspend our conscious awareness of.

Kind of like on an airliner when you're watching a really engrossing movie, and the plane enters some turbulence – but you don't notice until you take your headphones off and get up to go to the restroom.

Maybe these disturbances are good, maybe they're bad. Maybe they change moment to moment. Maybe they're why we have mood fluctuations, or an ability to excel in something one day, and we're a complete dufus the next. Maybe it's what the astrologers are working with when they say we're under the "influence of Mars" or "Uranus is in decline" (I think this has been my personal malady for several years now, but that's another subject.)

So much for the macro world. The problem is, the same spirals and circles and wheels within wheels are occurring in the micro world – the so-called "real" world – too, and at the same time. I recently heard a radio interview with the director of the National Institutes of Health, Dr. Elias Zerhouni, who made more or less in passing a profound statement: *"The [human] cell is more complex than the universe itself."* It goes without saying that if God is truly infinite, then that infinity goes 'down,' as well as 'up.'

So his creation Man isn't either small or large in the full scheme of things, and neither are the atoms that make up what we think of as our bodies. They're just somewhere (no-where?) in between "no-here" and "no-there" which bend around on each other and overlap into a never-ending circle of no-size. But that which we define as "real" ceases to exist somewhere along the way. Are we real or not? To paraphrase a recent president, it kinda depends on what your definition of "real" is.

Theoretical physicists have recently bridged that arbitrary gulf between existence and non-existence with string theory. Ironically, string theory was first described during the early days of Einstein, but not by him or any other physicist of the time, rather by suffragette, author and psychic Annie Besant.[14]

In casual terms, string theory postulates that the *actual* fundamental building blocks of the universe (supplanting the *previously-determined* fundamental building blocks of the universe) are little non-things going around in circles entering and leaving existence, and during the time they're "in" existence they are the bricks of the construction we call "us," and when they're not in existence maybe we aren't either, or if we are it's in a wholly different form (non-form?) than we think of as "ourselves." Kind of like motion picture film, which is comprised of 24 still pictures moving past a light each second, giving us the illusion of motion when there actually is none.

When you think about the fact that in any movie there is nearly as much "blank" time as picture time – as the shutter must be closed blocking the light while the film is pulled from frame to

---

[14] Besant and fellow clairvoyant Charles W. Leadbeater conducted a series of clairvoyant investigations of the inner workings of the atom. Their findings, with more than 200 drawings, closely parallel modern physics' understanding of string theory. See "Occult Chemistry" (Besant/Leadbeater, 1905).

frame – you've got a feeling for the true reality of our reality. As much non-matter time as matter time, as much non-reality as reality.

But for some reason, just as in the movie theater, we do not pay attention to that blank time, perhaps in part because not *all* of us is "blanking out" at the same time. In theater jargon this ignoring of what else is going on is called "suspension of disbelief." Maybe that's what we're doing every waking moment of our lives – suspending our acknowledgement that there's a whole lot more going on than we wish to be conscious of (teenagers do this quite well, you may have noticed). If our 'reality movie' gets really good, we blank everything out except it. We don't hear the phone, or our spouse talking to us, or even a police siren on the highway.

It is quite possible that somewhere down deep inside us – a place most of us rarely visit – we know more than we permit ourselves to consciously accept. With all the ghosts people apparently see, and the déjà vu that occurs on a regular basis, and the fact that more than two-thirds of us believe we have had "paranormal" experiences, maybe we're getting glimpses of this other half of our reality all the time, but don't know what to make of it, so we continue to ignore it. Like noticing a stranger's fly unzipped and turning away rather than saying something.

In order to go on about our life as we have learned to lead it, we must actually shut down a portion of our awareness and deny – based on what we think is lack of usefulness to our everyday situation – that blank period which completes the picture of our reality. And just as the 'empty space' in the universe is not empty at all, that blank period is not blank, but filled with goings-on which are every bit as real, important and interesting as that part we choose to see.

It is a universal desire to want to know who we really are and where we came from and what our relationship is to God and the Universe. Huge institutions have grown up over the centuries to give us answers. Maybe the answers to these questions lie in the blanked-out part of our reality. Certainly enough religions have tried to guide us to this place, and science isn't far behind.

So why don't we acknowledge it and find a way to go there? Maybe we're comfortable with life being what we perceive it to be, and we don't want anyone showing us another way. I remember my mother, at 50, comfortable in a religion whose take-it-or-leave-it tenets were set in stone around the turn of the 19th century, telling me she didn't want to hear any new theories of the Universe or God, because she didn't want to have to deal with the possibility that she'd been wrong all these years. She was also terrified she'd actually go to Hell if she started to really ask questions.

Many of us are like my mother, afraid of being aware of more than we have already accepted about reality, because we're uncomfortable with new information; it can destroy the set of references we've developed over the years for how we're supposed to deal with life. And then what would we do? "Don't question, it's not ours to know," "Don't upset the applecart," "Better leave well enough alone," were just a few of the rationalizations I constantly heard as a kid.

And of course there's the universal fear of the unknown: "Don't go into that dark forest, or you will surely die." Think Hansel & Gretel.

So we live in a half-lit world where we cannot see much of what's really going on – a dense forest filled with trees so large and incomprehensible that they block out the light. What we do see doesn't make much sense to us, and so we do the best we can, creating temporary explanations for everything while realizing inside they're not good enough. But we have nowhere to go for better answers. It's as if we're wandering in this forest, too afraid to seriously seek a way out. Just getting through the day without a monster eating us is the best we can hope for.

Mostly we tell ourselves that this stuff doesn't matter anyway, that we can get through life just fine without knowing any more than we know. Everything else is just academic dialogue anyway, we say, having nothing to do with practical reality.

Oh, sure, we had grand philosophical discussions in college, staying up half the night discussing why Siddhartha crossed the river, the relativistic nature of Aristotelian logic, and whether Kierkegaard and Sartre's existentialism really meant we were destined to be miserable all of our lives. But ever since the children arrived, or the job got intense, or the market tanked, or Mom moved in, the only thing we've been doing after midnight is trying to get half a night's sleep while worrying about getting through the next day. Like my mother, we just stopped thinking about it.

"Life's a sea of woes..."

We don't get through life very well. We have all kinds of problems and we have to work very hard to find the silver lining. In the half-light of limited consciousness in which we live, we believe that life is tough, and dangerous, and we just don't know what it's going to throw at us next. We've got to be girded for battle; people hurt us, strangers are dangerous, we get sick without warning, and most everything that happens to us is inexplicable. Most of us don't even really have the Devil to blame anymore, and the answer that "it's just God's Will" is not good enough either.

We savor the moments of happiness we have, because things are going to get worse, no matter what we think. Oh, yes, we may say "Every day in every way life is getting better and better," but we don't believe it. We grow old (if we don't get cancer at 30), get sick, lose our friends, and die. Life holds beautiful moments, it's true, but for most of us it is predominantly sad, scary, and out of our control. As Thoreau said, the majority of us lead lives of quiet desperation.

But that vast, mostly unexplored area of our being might hold some hope; that blank period, in between cycles of what we have been taught is the only reality. But how do we get at it? Where do we stand for the best view of what's really going on?

Religion attempts to get us there. From the earliest days, our religions have drawn us toward the "Light," as if light is God, and we as humans are far enough away from the Light to experience the woes of darkness: pain and suffering and fear (of the dark?). The implicit meaning is, "If we could only get to the Light, we would be made whole again."

Transcendental Meditation, indeed most forms of meditation, guide you to seek the light where you will find peace and tranquility…and transcendence from the mortal coil. Quakers, the religious movement that so greatly influenced the founding of the American nation, seek "the Light of God within," and before they adopted the name Quakers or even Friends they were called "Children of the Light."

There are variations of this theme throughout religion. From the earliest times, Christians have said "Christ is the Light of the World." Light has been a symbol of joy which dispelled the darkness of ignorance and fear. Lighting candles at Christmas (to symbolize Christ) followed in the tradition of earlier Roman and Hebrew customs. Candlemas, begun in the 5th Century, means literally "celebration of light," and has come to commemorate the presentation of Jesus in the Temple by his parents, when Simeon greeted him as "a light to lighten the Gentiles."

The word "light" is filled with hints to the secret of inner success. Light means "not dark." We cannot see in the dark, and seeing also means understanding. See? Light is bright…and "bright" also means intelligent. Intelligent's opposites include "dense" and "thick," while light is, well, "not dense"!

Light means "not heavy," which makes one think of floating on air – like angels? Like when you're so happy you're "walking on air"? And then there's "light in spirit," which is where we want to get to, isn't it?

But where is this light? It is across the dark forest, in the other half of our reality – the blank part, the non-physical half – where string theory takes us when it's not matter; where religion and meditation and other "paths to the Light" bid us travel.

◊

"But then one sees that not even the quality of being (if that may be called a "quality") belongs to what is described. It is a <u>possibility</u> for being or a <u>tendency</u> for being."
  - Werner Heisenberg

p 44, *Physics and Philosophy: The Revolution in Modern Science*,
Copyright 1958 by Werner Heisenberg.
Reprinted by permission of HarperCollins Publishers

Chapter V: Intention, Our Fundamental Reality

In acting classes, the teacher will often ask the student, "What is your *intention* in this scene?" The way a character in a play or movie becomes real to an audience and interacts with others in the story as a fully-formed, believable person is not just determined by the words in the script, but by the inner intention the actor chooses for that character in any given part of a scene. What does the character believe about himself, the other characters, about life, about the situation he finds himself in?

What does she really want, down deep, as a foundation beneath the words she's saying, in each scene, and in the story overall?

Just as in life where our real but hidden, subtextual intentions permeate our words – often revealing in spite of ourselves that we're lying or attempting to manipulate, a character's intention is conveyed to the audience as subtext which makes the character come alive. Actors know this, and choose their characters' intentions carefully in preparation for a role.

The importance of intention is often illustrated to new acting students by having them read a section of dialogue from a scene over and over, each time choosing a totally different intention for the character. The same lines read with different intentions will come out of an actor's mouth with different inflections, different emphasis, and with totally different subtextual emotions, all based on the character's underlying intention.

Oh, you say, that's fine for acting…but what does it have to do with real life? Everything. No less a sage than Will Shakespeare reminds us that "All the world's a stage, and all the men and women merely players…" Our intention in every moment is sensed by others, no matter how they wish to deny that it's so.

There's another acting truism: "Acting is reacting." So is living. How do we react to events that occur? We react out of our intention, and our intention is based on what we believe. And our beliefs are shaped first from what we are taught – and second, NOT from the experiences we have had, but rather how we have reacted to those experiences.

Werner Erhardt, the founder of the '70s psychological phenomenon *est*, said that the hardest thing in life to do is to approach each new experience as in fact a NEW experience, not colored or distorted by our feelings about any previous experiences, however similar. The moment we let our conclusions from earlier bad experiences color our expectations, allowing the new experience to stand alone is almost impossible.

Several years ago, I made a documentary film on hunger in America. During the production, my crew and I discovered a family of five living in their car in upscale Santa Monica, parked on a street where ironically the typical house was valued at well above the average middle class home of its time. Out of gas and money, the four adults and a 13-year old child had been in the car for five weeks, and during this whole time no one on the entire block had ever ventured out to see what was going on. But that's another story.

When I showed up with my film crew and ask them to talk to us, the youngest adult in the family, age 32, and the most likely to be employable, was clearly in a state of almost deranged detachment. His eyes were wide and glassy and his skittish demeanor gave us the feeling that he might at any second bolt and run or just stop talking to us. This was not a man you would consider hiring for a job.

Yet as we became acquainted with him and his family's story of how they fell on hard times, we began to see that this was not his normal personality. They had arrived from Ohio, the two adult men with long-distance offers of jobs from acquaintances in LA. A recession was rocking the eastern half of the U.S., so like the star-crossed Jodes in Steinbeck's *Grapes of Wrath*, they had packed up their belongings, bought a small trailer to tow behind their car, and set out for California – the promised land. (Out of a deep sense of irony developed during production, we titled the documentary *Hunger in the Promised Land*.)

Somewhere in Texas their trailer was stolen, and in Arizona their car broke down, requiring an expensive 'take-it-or-leave-it' repair job in the desert. Arriving in Los Angeles, almost out of money, they contacted their job connections, only to discover that the economic downturn had hit here, too. There weren't any jobs for them, after all. In this era before cell phones, their friends had not been able to get in touch with them to advise them not to come.

For a time, they took refuge in a cheap motel while the men went out job hunting. The father was 60, he'd been a truck driver, and worked on air conditioners from time to time. But now no one was hiring, or those who had openings chose younger people to fill the job.

The 32-year-old son, a carpenter's helper, had no contacts in the area, so he began answering any and all kinds of unskilled labor ads, offering to sweep floors or carry out trash for a little money to feed his family. After a time he didn't even ask for money in exchange for his work, just food.

No matter, at each interview he was turned down, and the family's situation became more desperate, until finally they could no longer afford the motel and took to sleeping in their car, hoping that the next day would bring their salvation. The longer they stayed in the car, the longer they went without the ability to wash themselves and change their clothes, adding to an already impossible situation.

Too proud to ask for handouts, unable to get welfare or food stamps because they had no permanent mailing address, they began raiding dumpsters behind grocery stores.

The adult son bore the pressure of the family's dire straits, realizing his father wasn't going to be able to find work. It was then that his *intention* changed, from offering his services as a capable employee to desperately needing to find food and shelter for his family. This desperation showed clearly on his face each time he walked into a store and asked for work. It affected his mannerisms, his speech, his expectations, and the results he got.

We saw it, and it scared us. Clearly no one was going to hire him now, and his situation – their situation – was becoming graver by the day.

My crew and I could not remain detached observers for long. We pooled some money and found the family a motel room nearby, bought them food and gas for their car, and several of us made calls to help them find jobs. Two days after they moved into the motel, took showers, washed their clothes and got a couple good nights' sleep, this family of Jodes became relaxed and coherent again.

The glaze in the older son's eyes disappeared, the frantic tightness in his face relaxed, and he smiled for the first time. The 13-year-old boy who had sat mute in the back of the car laughed and played with us. Just knowing they had emotional support allowed them to become 'civil' again in job interviews.

Within a week, both father and son had found work. Once again their intention had changed from desperation to basic human need... still tough to deal with, but at least one that allows most people to reach out without feeling they're going to get their hand bitten.

We stayed in touch with our new friends for awhile, and when we last heard from them, a year later, they were managing a motel in Long Beach, the boy was in school, and all were doing fine.

What we believe – we call it "know" – about ourselves and about the world is, for all intents and purposes, true. Because even if it's not, we will act as though it is, and that's the experience we're going to have. All other possibilities will be blocked or ignored.

We are all little universes, literally spinning our own complex reality. We have arrived at our own personal conclusions about the world we are in. Just as people throughout history have thought that they understood the world, God, and the universe, we think that we know how life is. If someone disagrees too much with us, we know deep inside that they're probably misinformed, uneducated, or simply wrong.

But that's only a convenience we tell ourselves. Beneath that comfortable exterior, our own concept of our universe is changing slightly every moment. Like the ripples from two stones dropped in the water, when the energy patterns from our reality bump up against those of someone else, we both change ever so slightly.

You've heard the saying, "When a butterfly flaps its wings in China, Chicago experiences a windstorm," making the point that a single ripple, arriving from an event in a life halfway around the world, will change our concept of reality in some infinitesimal way.

We can deny this shift, and try to shut it out, but some part of us experiences it. Subtle perceptual shifts are like seeds, they may lie dormant for years before taking root, but they are there. Multiply them by the billions of such ripples that enter our awareness every day, and we begin to have some idea of the transitory nature of our perception of reality.

> *- Yesterday we believed the earth was the center of the universe.*
>
> *- Yesterday we believed that the earth was flat.*
>
> *- Yesterday we believed that man could not fly.*
>
> *- Yesterday we believed that man could not run a mile in less than four minutes.*
>
> *- Yesterday we believed our body was our unknowable enemy – an evil twin which would cause us greater and greater discomfort before killing us completely.*
>
> *- But this is Today.*

◊

Chapter VI: The Great I AM

How is it that trapeze artists and soldiers and dancers and sports players and *Cirque de Soleil* performers can put their bodies through rigors that would send most of us quickly to the hospital? How can they run and jump and dive into the ground and crawl under barbed wire and tumble and careen into each other and still pick themselves up and go on as if nothing happened?

Training, we're told. Clearly that training includes the understanding and adaptation of their minds to the unusual stresses and pressures they are going to experience, so nothing seems unexpected when it happens. It is the unexpected that hurts us. They do not experience the fear that you and I would if we were to do the same thing, because our muscles and our ligaments…and our minds…are not comfortable with what's happening – they're scared.

And it's that fear that causes us to be hurt.

Ever notice that drunks, children and small animals survive car wrecks a lot more often than us "normal" people? Why? They're not afraid. Take a tumble you're not ready for, freeze and try to prevent it (especially if your decorum is at stake), and you're in for a torn muscle or broken bone. Relax as it's happening, imagine you're a football player getting tackled in a fun game, and you'll often come up unscathed.

I was lucky once, when I sailed off the front of a motorcycle going 40 mph, back in the days of "who needs a helmet?" An inexperienced rider trying to see Europe on the cheap, I had rented a bike I had no business trying to ride and wound up locking up the front brake while trying to slow down on the rocky shoulder of a narrow French highway. The front wheel stopped abruptly but not me, I kept going, right between the handlebars.

The last thing I remember was hitting the rocks with my hands, then tucking my shoulder and tumbling onto the side of this two-lane road.

Somehow I had instinctively fallen into a "tuck and roll," as if this was something I had been doing forever, and that saved my life. Apparently my mind, seeking a reference for what was happening, grabbed onto the memory of this maneuver. It could have been from childhood days of playground football, or maybe from something I had learned in the Army, the "run, lunge and roll."

Wherever it came from, the instinct took over at the critical moment and saved me. I was out cold for 18 minutes, but survived with only a body full of bruises and cuts I thought would never heal. God only knows what would have happened if I had braced up in terror as I flew through the air.

Left to its own devices, the mind often seems to know better what to do than "we" do. But what's the difference between "it" and "me"?

In 1926 Ernest Holmes wrote the famous book *The Science of Mind*, in which he presented a new approach to spirituality, health and one's relationship to God. He believed that in spite of the magnificent potential life presents to us, that life can be only what we believe it to be. In Holmes' words, *"our belief sets the limit to our demonstration of a Principle which, of Itself, is without limit."*

Holmes suggested that if God, the center and source of all, is omnipotent (all power), omniscient (all knowing), and omnipresent (everywhere), then we must be in actual fact a manifestation of God. But even though we have that vast potential inside us, we become only what we think we can become, and we know as reality only what we think we know as reality. Whatever else is possible within us, children of the "all things are possible" God, cannot become real in our lives because we will not permit it!

God cannot manifest something into our world which we cannot accept, for even if it were to manifest, our minds wouldn't let us perceive it; we would ignore it or refuse to believe it. Mostly it's the latter, in my experience. How many times have we been shown an unbelievable something and walked away looking for a reason why it couldn't be true? You can't imagine how many years it took me to actually believe that I was actually doing "remote viewing." No matter how often I was right, I knew in my heart I was just a "good guesser." I couldn't accept that I might be a "psychic" – whatever that was.

It took me an equally long time to accept that the techniques described in this book actually work. We too often ascribe these mystifying things to something we must have imagined, or worse, to the work of the Devil.

My father used to tell me that I was doing something evil by dabbling in psychic things. But his father used to tell him that the radio was an instrument of Satan and that God would never let man reach the moon. His father probably told him that God would never let man fly, and *his* father probably told him that you'd die if you traveled over 30 miles per hour. What are we telling our children today that will be fodder for jokes fifty years from now?

According to Ernest Holmes, if we are to change anything about us, from our feelings to our experiences to our health; if we are to begin to have an unimaginably different kind of life, we must begin by "changing our mind" about what is possible, and we must do so completely and entirely, *even in the face of no evidence*. The Bible says, "All things are possible to those who love the Lord," but very few of us actually believe it for ourselves, down deep inside.

If we really accept that all things are possible, wouldn't it be nice to start with the possibility of a healthier life? To do so we must begin to play at allowing new possibilities, possibilities beyond where our present thinking will permit us to go, knowing that as we expand our thinking to allow new possibilities, perhaps they can then become real to us.

Put another way, the new 'it' may already be there all the time, but we won't see it until we know we can. Which, ironically, is exactly what the Bible and the physicist are both telling us about the true nature of reality. In one case, "Ask and ye shall receive," and in the other, "The observer's expectations affect the outcome of the experiment."

Christians call this faith. But while Holmes taught that Jesus was the Christ incarnate, the perfect manifestation of a perfect God, he also taught that we are all perfect manifestations of a perfect God, and that the difference between us and Christ is simply our relative lack of understanding – and our incorrect (re)actions as a result – of who and what we really are: children of God.

In the 1930s and '40s, the era when patients went to hospitals and sanitariums for "treatment" for illness, Holmes taught spiritual "treatment" as a technique for changing one's life (spiritual healing), and for physical healing as well, since both forms of healing are merely different aspects of the whole self. Science of Mind "practitioners" learned that *dis*-ease often manifests from our lack of ease (stress) endured over a long period of time.

Modern medicine concurs. But Holmes went further, arguing that health is our natural state, and this health lies beneath the mistaken appearance of disease. But because we do not know this, we cannot move out of our experience of dis-ease. God cannot give us that which we cannot accept. And if we, like my late grandmother, only accept that we are sick and never that we can get completely well, we can never be healed. Ironically, it is our free will which binds us. Our thinking frequently leaves us believing life is terrible, when it's possible that it's only our thinking that's terrible. "Stinking thinking," as one Science of Mind minister used to call it.

Once again, it brings to mind the evangelist's question as he has his hand on the Sister's head: "Do you believe God can heal you?" The answer must be "Yes" or no healing can occur. And then the question follows, "Do you know God *has* healed you?" This is the very determiner of who stays healed and who doesn't. How much do they believe, *know* beyond a shadow of a doubt, that they are really healed?

Holmes offered a phrase to help keep the mind from closing down in fear when something bad happens: "Not a word of truth to it." If you stub your toe, in that split second before you make a tight face and screech in pain, relax and say, "Not a word of truth to it. I thought it was going to hurt, but amazingly, it doesn't!" You'll probably have to do this several times, in the face of no evidence, (another pet Holmes phrase) but you'll be surprised at how much less pain you'll have than you expected.

After a few tries at it, you may even discover that there really IS no pain from some bang or scrape or cut which used to hurt like hell. Then you might want to tackle a book written by Raymond Charles Barker entitled *Treat Yourself to Life*, before moving on to the richer but denser *Science of Mind*, which can occupy your bedside table for years into the future.

The Power of The Word

"In The Beginning Was The Word...And The Word Was God." John 1:1. What does this mean? Doesn't it mean that the most powerful force in the universe, outside of the maker of that universe itself, was and is the WORD; the intelligent noise of the universe, the inspired reverberation of the atoms and molecules one upon the other, and even, at our level of reality, The Spoken Word, speech?

What is speech? The noisy culmination and result of a terrifically complex combination of activities in the universe: atoms and molecules moving with precision within the organs of our bodies, merged with and guided by (non-physical) thought – conscious and subconscious; then nerves and muscles dancing together in a symphony of harmonic activity, moving upon the breath to form Something out of Nothing. Formless air molded by our thoughts to yield substance and meaning, emanating from us at frequencies which may be perceived and translated by other beings like us, and understood to mean something far more than the sum of their actions and vibrations! An amazing power! Reminds me of radio transmissions – something out of nothing.

According to the Bible, Jesus said, *"As a man thinketh in his heart, so is he."* That is, we speak and act from our *intention* (!) and our intention arises from what we believe in our heart. Could it be that he was trying to tell us that the spoken word is the most powerful thing in the universe? That every word out of our mouth has the power to bind us or set us free, to change the way we think and feel...and are...for better or worse.

In the Pentateuch, Moses asks God who he is, and God answers, *"I Am that I Am."* Well if God is the master and creator of all, and he is the big "I Am," and if we were made in the image and likeness of God, then are we "little 'I ams' "? If so, no wonder most of us think life's so rotten:

"I am sick and tired..."

"I am so broke..."

"I am so stressed..."

"I am fed up with..."

"I am about to blow my stack..."

"I am always in pain..."

"I am..."

These are little spins we're constantly putting into reality, which come back to define for us who we are. But we don't notice ourselves creating them, we just notice them after they've had time to culture and grow. "Yikes, look at my poor situation," we observe, not remembering that it was us who might very well have created it with our sacred and powerful Word.

Now you can buy an app for your phone which analyzes the voice patterns of people you're near, listening to their subtext – their intention – while you're hearing the specific words themselves. (As if we can't already tell when someone's lying.)

If you've ever had your handwriting analyzed, you know that certain patterns seem to reflect certain personality traits – patterns in the way you think of yourself. Police departments use such analysis to test for criminal predilections. Analysts also tell you that to change those traits in yourself, start by changing the way you write.

Changing the way you think of your universe may be just as easy…it starts by just changing the things you say. Your words might be the key to changing yourself completely.

What if it were that simple. Wouldn't it be just like the Maker of the Universe to put the key to our health and happiness right in front of our faces!

This isn't new stuff. Not only has the Bible tried to teach it to us, but many ancient and venerated books call upon us to speak that which we wish to be true about ourselves. Protestant "salvation" offers it if you will only believe – "speak that Christ is your savior," they say. The Buddha instructed the listener to "speak only well of oneself and of others." Ben Franklin said the same thing. Each put it in a slightly different way, addressing a culture in the terms that culture understood, but they all made the entreaty – the instruction – that he who would live in the light of God, or in Nirvana, or experience the joy of heaven in his life, must first know that he is "already there." The difficulty in understanding this is lodged in our concept of Time. We'll get into that later.

I've always been fascinated with the Bible's account of the teaching of Jesus, that little children would have an easier time of understanding his message than adults. As if we grownups are looking for something complex, rare, and hard to attain, and so ignore the simple, beautiful answers that are right at our feet. We seem to take Jesus' simple message and twist it and turn it and convolute it and analyze it until it takes an opus the size of the old New York City phone book to make it understandable (?) to adults. And then, of course, it takes a cadre of "very wise and learnéd men" to translate it for us. St. Augustine spent a lifetime at it, so did Thomas Aquinas and so many more. Is it really that hard to understand?

Making things complicated is a universal human foible. It's the same thing that happens when the government takes over childcare or street sweeping. Well-meaning people create institutions which become heavy on bureaucracy and administration (because it's easier to make and interpret policy about something than to actually do that thing). Then of course the priorities become skewed. Administrators and bureaucrats become more concerned with keeping and enhancing their own jobs than with actually putting policies into action. Added interpretations are handed down, constricting even more those who are trying to deliver the actual service intended by the institution, and finally the result is that hardly any of the originally intended benefit actually trickles down to the people it was intended for.

Oh, I'm not pointing fingers. I've been there and done that. You probably have, too. It's human nature, but it's something we must be aware of, and fight.

Speaking of simple answers right at our feet, many nutritionists have come to the conclusion that one of the very best sources of the vitamins and minerals the body needs for optimum health – delivered in a pH balance closest to that of blood (so the body takes it up completely with the least effort) – is found in probably the most ubiquitous plant on our planet: grass. The variation most palatable to the western sugar- and carbohydrate-conditioned palate is common wheat grass, the stuff cows munch on for days on end, and eventually make milk – and steaks – from. (Yes, there's kale, and quinoa, and even chocolate...but...)

An acquired taste for most, to be sure, but wheat grass juice is a primary food source used by some health centers that deal with terminally ill cancer patients, because it gives the most complete nourishment for the least amount of energy spent digesting it.

Grass! Oops, we've been so close all this time! It's that *other* kind of weed, growing under our noses! And it's been there since the beginning of time. Maybe there's a lot more right under our noses that we're missing, too, because we're looking for something difficult, complex and sophisticated, when the answer is so simple.

Maybe we missed *this* simple truth, too: maybe the key to our health is in our mouth. Maybe our words have the power to heal us. We know they can "turn away wrath." We know they can "soothe the savage breast." We know our soft words can take away a baby's fear and pain...and an adult's, too. When Jack Houck touched my forehead and said "You've just forgotten," I was healed. They were just words, spoken with specific intention, but they worked.

But remember the second part: I had to accept the healing. If I had not truly *known* and *accepted* that I was healed, and let go of all my ideas and beliefs about learned doctors and diagnoses and the irreversibility of diseases like that, I would have just thanked him for his kind words and gone on worrying about my eye. Or the spider web would have come back in a week. The fact that I did not do that is the key to the effectiveness of the process.

So the Word is *speaking* and *knowing* together. When the Creator speaks, there is no possibility of doubt in the words. When we speak our healing, those words also must be spoken with the understanding that it has happened, it is done. We are changing the future, after all.

There are many and varied beliefs as to how and why this works, but it works nevertheless. I don't need to know how an automobile runs to enjoy taking it out for a drive.

But here's my belief about it anyway, to add to your collection:

In the Bible, God tells Moses, "I am that I am." There's a good start, right there. What am I? I am what I declare myself to be, sick or healthy, injured or healed, happy or sad. But this does not happen all at once. Often, because the manifestation of that declaration arrives late, we lose faith before it arrives. We get up from being healed and say, "Hey, I don't see any change, it must have not worked." Remember what Scarlett Johansson's "Lucy" said in the movie by Luc Besson: "The thought has to move through time!"

Give it time!

Hey! For God's sake, even Jesus took the weekend to rise from the dead! How is it you expect instant results in your case? When the doctor gives us a prescription and says, "Take these for 10 days," do you expect to be well tomorrow? No! Not on day one, or even a week later most times! Why must other kinds of healing be demonstrated immediately or they're not valid?

Elsewhere in the Bible we're told that God is *"All in All,"* and *"the kingdom of heaven is within,"* and *"nothing is that was not made by God."* It seems pretty clear that someone is trying to make the point that everything comes from, and is, God.

So, wait. If God is everywhere, then is God in me? It must be so, or else you have to do some fancy semantical dancing (well, is God omnipresent, or not?). And if God is everywhere, then God must be in all of me (is God All in All, or not?). Not only in all of me...oh, oh, now take a breath:

If God is in all of me, and God is everywhere...

(okay, remember now, this is *my* concept, you don't have to accept it to learn to help heal yourself, but you did ask…)

…what part of me isn't God?

We've always had a lot of trouble there, haven't we? Lots of issues crop up here. We just can't reconcile our feeling of worthlessness and just plain stupidity (plus the fact that someone told us we were born into Original Sin) with the concept clearly set forth in many sacred books that we are made from God-stuff in God's image. Period.

The answer has to be: No part of me <u>isn't</u> the stuff of God! I'm *all* God…not all *of* God, to be sure, but all of me is God stuff, or God isn't all the stuff in the universe after all. But it isn't "I AM GOD and YOU'RE nothing!" It's rather, "I am not some outrageously egotistical special individual, I am merely a manifestation of God in the physical – the thought of God moving through time. Just as the tree, the animal, the rock, the star, the universe itself – and you – are different manifestations of the maker, the great I AM.

What if…what if I accept the possibility that God is in me and is me, and as such I AM the creator of my universe, just as God is the creator of the entire Universe. And as God thinks the Universe into being, then is not my universe, my reality, created out of my thought?

All this time I've been thinking that I <u>observe</u> what I am, that it exists before I think about it, and then I state what I observe. What if it's the other way around? What if, like Heisenberg's observer-affecting-the-experiment conclusion, *that which I observe* is there only because of what I *think* I see? Kind of like a beautiful woman who slithers into a sexy dress only to look in the mirror and see nothing except fat hips. What if she decided her hips were perfect? Would they suddenly become perfect? And in whose eyes? There are lots of sexy women whose hips are wider than the American cultural ideal. They don't seem to care. In their universe, they're just right. And you know what? When they think so, others think so, too. And if they don't, they're not noticed! But the day that same woman spends her time at a party worrying about the size of her hips, everyone sees a completely different woman – in the same body. *Thoughts create reality.*

We are not very good observers, because our observation is affected by too much experience, and experience is pretty much based on what we perceive on the physical side of our existence – what "happens" to us. We can't see who we really are anymore. We can only see what we think we have become, or what we're afraid others think of us. It seems that only little children can easily see truth. *"Lest ye become like a little child ye cannot enter the kingdom of heaven."* Maybe the real truth is, we are in fact all quite wonderful children of God – another way of saying "manifestations" of God – underneath it all. We just have to refocus our attention away from all the bad stuff we've decided prevents us from experiencing that joy and that ability to regain and maintain our good health.

Consider this: we know that a house is built by the mind. What? Yes. It is first *dreamed* up, *thought* about, *contemplated*. The architect *thinks* about it, then draws it – as the thought guides the hand. The builder reads and understands the drawings, and considers – in his mind – how to make these ideas manifest in physical reality. The Maker may have created the raw materials – stone, wood, metal – which the builder uses, but the house is built first in the mind, and then, over time, manifested in the physical.

Did you ever have an idea for a project and then have someone tell you it can't be done? You either believed him and quit, or you believed yourself and continued to look for someone who agreed with you that it could be done.

There are people who live their lives with this concept: I AM what I think I am. Life is what I think it is…in the face of no evidence. Most of the time we call these people crazy. Whose definition is that? Not theirs.

Crazy People Aren't So Bad!

Wilbur and Orville Wright were crazy. They didn't just walk down to Kitty Hawk in 1903 and suddenly fly their airplane. They spent years, thousands of hours, on those cold, empty dunes of North Carolina, every day putting the idea of an airplane (they had thought up, talked about, drawn on paper, then built) on its rails, pulling it by hand along the hard-packed sand into the biting wind, only to have each attempt fail, devastatingly – for years. They suffered frostbite, sunstroke, infections from insect bites and numerous injuries. They had little food, less shelter, and endured the jeers and jokes of everyone around them. Not only did Americans scoff at them, they were the laughing stock of all of France, too. "*Bluffeurs,*" the French called them; two small-town boys who couldn't possibly fly.

They wanted to give up in 1901, two years before they would be successful even once. Returning from months of bruising and dangerous experiments, Orville wrote his sister that "man will not fly for a thousand years." The US government was spending millions on the best scientists and engineers to build a successful flying machine. Alexander Graham Bell invested his large ego and an equally large fortune trying to do it. But the two crazy bicycle repairmen from Dayton did not give up. They knew they had a plane that would fly, even though it existed for years only in their mind. Every day when they went out into the blowing sand to try again, their aeroplane was already flying – in their mind. And every day that the physical one crashed, leaving them with more bruises and broken bones, they got up and tried again. Crazy men.

I AM.

Jim Carrey tells the story of his years as a mediocre comic, getting poorly-paying gigs at mediocre clubs around Los Angeles while watching the Jerry Seinfelds and Jay Lenos and David

Lettermans of the comedy world (who started only a few years earlier than he did) achieve fame and fortune.

He says that late at night he would go up to the top of Mulholland Drive on the rim of the Santa Monica Mountains overlooking LA, find a secluded area and walk to the edge of the mountain. Then he would take out of his pocket a check, made out to himself for ten million dollars. He would pantomime receiving this check from a studio head, and thanking the man for it. Then he would look out across the lights of the city and declare at the top of his lungs[15], "I AM THE FUNNIEST COMIC ALIVE. I AM PAID TEN MILLION DOLLARS PER MOVIE! I AM A STAR!" He says he did this until he could actually, completely believe it. He carried that check in his back pocket and acted out that scenario for more than ten years. Jim Carrey was crazy? You might have thought so.

I AM.

The actor and comedian Billy Crystal told an audience recently that for years in New York, while he was trying to succeed as a comic, his joint tax return with his wife showed less than $4,000 in income, and half of that was from his substitute teaching jobs. In spite of that, he knew he was going to be a successful comic.

Seven years later, he still never doubted he would be successful, even after his managers refused to let him accept a job on the premiere season of "Saturday Night Live" because they thought he was not ready. Not even ready for "late night," after seven years. Seven more years later he finally achieved fame and fortune, but all the while, during more than 15 years of struggle, he never doubted that he would be enormously successful. He feared…but he never doubted.

---

[15] Note: *Out loud!*

Fifteen years, in the face of very little evidence.

WHAT ARE YOU?

What does this have to do with healing, you ask? Well what is the first question the faith healer asks? "Do you believe you can be healed?" First, heal the mind.

You've seen this little experiment before in other contexts. Let's try it again, this time for the sake of our health:

Take a pad of paper and a pencil and complete the following sentence:

"I am _____."

Do it as many times as you get answers, and write all of your answers down, all the good, the bad, the ugly. Be brutally honest, no one is going to read this but you.

Then look at what you have written. Consider the person who is all of these things. Do you like them? Do you respect them? What would you change?

So, you have just declared what you know to be true. You have described yourself in your personal universe. Not *the* Universe, but the one you live in. Remember, you're not *The Creator*, you're *a* creator. Do you understand that this is only one of the possible realities you can experience? You can change your mind at any time, and since the future isn't here yet, alter that future.

Knowing that "I AM" is such powerful medicine, you can, like Jim Carrey, make a statement of "fact" using what you would like to be true, and amazingly, by practicing every day – "in the face of no evidence" – you will see the change gradually begin to occur.

Or maybe you won't. Sometimes these things happen all at once – very long after you've started. Physicists call this the quantum aspect of reality. On the quantum (sub-atomic) level, and thus in reality, energy does not build or diminish linearly, in a smooth, imperceptibly gradual way, like we think of it. As power is added, it remains at one strength level for some time, then "jumps" to the next level instantaneously, then plateaus for awhile, and jumps again to the next level. We notice it when we're learning something new – it's hard for a long time, and seems like we're not learning anything, then, all of a sudden, just about the time we've given up, we "get it," and move to the next level. Many things work this way, losing weight, toning our bodies, learning to ride a bike, or land an airplane.

Changing your life works the same way.

A trivial personal example: When I was 20, and out in the 'real world' for the first time, away from my small-town American roots, I looked at myself and realized that I was a classic nerd, capital N. During high school I had successfully hidden myself away from teen social life by being consumed by electronics and amateur radio. I could turn on the powerful short-wave radio in my basement and carry on lengthy conversations with people around the world, but put me in the soda shop/teen club where the other high school kids hung out and I was suddenly mute. The word Wallflower was invented for me – I stood against the wall during high school dances, hoping it hid me.

In college, when I did get up the nerve to ask girls out, they typically found an excuse not to go. "I'm washing my hair tonight" was one frequently used reason (yes, there was a time before hair dryers!). The less-imaginative ones just said, "Sorry, I'm busy," or "I don't date…" politely leaving off the rest of the sentence: "…you."

By 20, I was sick of failure. I wanted to be like those cool, successful guys who seemed always to be dressed well, and always had a come-hither smile for the ladies – which worked. I had heard my father say that these kind of people were really no different than us. "They all put their pants on one leg at a time," he'd say.

So I decided to try something new. Very secretly, for fear of being found out and made more fun of, I would look myself in the mirror every morning and – no matter what I actually saw – would say, "Ben, you are a good looking guy, you dress well, and I don't know why, but girls really like you." Then I would pinch a zit, adjust my nerdy glasses and head off to class, hoping no one had overheard.

I did this for years, never telling a soul, never being discovered, with not much changing, either. But I didn't care. It became a habit, out of bed, shower, teeth brushed, shave, get dressed, talk to myself in the mirror. It wasn't a 'pep talk' – "Today you're going to really knock 'em dead…" It was just what someone in the '70s started calling an "affirmation." Yes, you're right, a variation of Al Franken's 'Stuart Smalley' character on Saturday Night Live: "I'm good enough, I'm smart enough, and by golly, people like me!"

Along about the fourth year I started dating attractive, interesting women. By year six, I was in New York City, occasionally getting dates with actresses and models. (Well, I didn't ask for *wisdom*, I just said I wanted to be attractive to women.)

What began as a lie told to myself every day in the face of the sad truth of my situation, gradually filtered down into my subconscious and was accepted. Somehow apparently this is the way it works. First comes the "I am," and then the manifestation follows. And remember, it may take a long time.

Playing this interesting game of lying to yourself in the arena of interpersonal relationships is one thing, but we're afraid it can become dangerous when we try it with physical things.

During the Silva classes, we were given interesting homework. Late one rainy afternoon in our classroom in midtown Manhattan, we were told that when we left the class, to start to walk home, and, playing the game we were learning in class, 'call' a cab – just with our mind. The next day we were to report how many blocks it took us to get one.

This was the time before Uber and Lyft, and anyone who'd spent any time in New York City knew you couldn't find a cab at rush hour in Midtown, much less in the rain, so common sense said that this was an impossible task. But we had agreed to play the game all the way to the end, and these were today's instructions.

I'll never forget that day. It was a Friday afternoon just after five o'clock when we left the class. It was still pouring outside. I raised my umbrella and walked two blocks in the direction of my apartment across town. It was going to be a long walk. There wasn't an empty cab in sight – and at least a dozen people were standing on the street waiting to fight for the first one.

Oh, well. I started the internal process, "creating the possibility" in my mind that a cab would not only be available, but, what the heck, it would pull up to the curb, the door would open, and I would step inside without breaking stride. Why not! It was possible. Not very likely, but I had to admit, it could happen.

I hunched my shoulders against the rain, strode on, and got into the game, now imagining a full-blown image of this impossible scene. At least I wasn't thinking about how wet my shoes were getting. A block later I was crossing Park Avenue, oblivious to everything but the imaginary film playing out in my mind, when a taxi pulled to a stop 50 feet ahead of me and a woman opened the door to get out.

My heart quickened, my mouth probably dropped open. As I approached, my impulse was to run for the cab, in case others were running, too. But I refused to look around, and deliberately maintained my pace. The woman paid her fare, opened her umbrella, and stepped out. Seeing me approaching, she left the door open. I got in the cab, sat down, and laughed hysterically. It had taken less than four blocks.

I used that technique for decades afterward.

One of the other games we played was keeping razor blades sharp. We had been experimenting with imagining going "inside" metals and rocks and plants, and sensing what it felt like. A lot of us used razors for shaving, and the instructor suggested that since razor blades were just formed pieces of metal, and the sharp edges were merely an arrangement of molecules, we might want to try and imagine the molecules keeping their formation longer than normal, or reforming, if they were knocked askew by the act of coming against the molecules of a beard.

Why not? For the next several weeks, we played that game, imagining our razor blades' edge molecules staying in sharp formation. Some of the students decided that putting them into a particular box at night would help. The box was imagined to sharpen the blades overnight. Most of our blades lasted three or four times longer than normal.

We played the same game with batteries, and eventually with the plants most New Yorkers keep just above the threshold of death in their apartments. Hey, the most successful gardeners talk to their plants, after all.

It was all fun, and most surprisingly, it was successful. Our plants blossomed, batteries lasted longer, and even parking spots miraculously became available around town when we needed them. In Manhattan! No kidding.

Once, years later in Los Angeles, I was a partner in a successful documentary production company, and I wanted to fire a troublesome, argumentative employee. Problem was, I knew the guy would throw a huge fit and maybe even cause legal trouble if I did. Pondering the problem with my partner over a beer one night,

I determined that I would "do that thing I did" and imagine a future in which the employee quit. Sitting there, I said, "I create the possibility that Mr. X is going to walk into my office and say, 'I'm really sorry, Ben, but I'm going to have to quit, something better has come up for me.' " Once again, why not?

"When?" my partner asked.

"Within three weeks, I imagined aloud.

Next day at the office, our secretary came in, furious at how he was being treated by Mr. X, and I confided to him what I had done. He shrugged, and said, "I wish you'd just fire him." I asked him to be patient and see what happens.

You already know the end of the story. On a Monday morning two weeks later, the employee in question stepped into my office and announced with great sadness that he was going to have to resign. Somebody had offered him a job he just couldn't refuse! My assistant overheard, and stepped in behind him to watch, grinning from ear to ear.

I don't know *how* it's done – that part's none of my business, but I know *that* it works, and I'm for sure not the only one who can do it.

◊

Casual Magic

Canadian television personality Maria LeRose was five months pregnant with her first child when she started bleeding – a bad sign at any stage of pregnancy. Her husband rushed her to the doctor, who confirmed by ultrasound that the fetus was still alive, and advised them that extreme care would have to be taken to make sure it survived to term. She was told to go home and spend the remaining four months flat on her back in bed, or else she'd lose the baby.

Maria was an active young woman, a successful television journalist, and the prospect of lying in bed for the next 120 days straight sounded more like a prison sentence than anything else. But she wanted the baby, so at home her husband tucked her in for a real "long winter's nap" and went off to work.

As she tells it, Maria sifted through her mind, looking for some way to accept this enforced inactivity, and then she drifted into a kind of quiet, prayerful meditative state, asking her body to tell her what was wrong and help her heal it. She says that suddenly she felt like she was shrinking, and found herself flowing through her body wearing kind of a scuba suit.

As she moved through her body, she came upon an area that was bleeding – a kind of a tear in a membrane somewhere. She stopped, and calmly *began to caress the wound, soothing and healing it. After a time, she realized that the bleeding had stopped, the wound was closed and healed. She says she "absolutely knew" the tear in her womb was healed. Then she fell asleep.*

Several hours later, her husband returned home and she woke up. As he entered the room, he looked at her and his mouth dropped open. "What have you done?" he asked her. "There's a glow about you that sure wasn't there when I left. Something has happened." She smiled and shared her experience with him.

After that day, Maria did not stay in her bed, she did not bleed again, and she gave birth to a healthy daughter four months later. Ironically, she did not think about using that miraculous technique for anything else in her life until I mentioned to her that I was writing this book.

Chapter VII: What If? - Making New Metaphors

So if we can call cabs in the rain, and make razor blades last longer, and make spoons bend just by yelling at them; if at least half of our existence is in the blank periods between "beingnesses," obviously we have to consider the possibility that we don't know everything there is to know about "What it is, what it was, and what it shall be," to quote late comedian Robin Williams.

Putting religion, science and philosophy aside, let's Lighten Up. Consider this:

What if the "I" as we think of ourselves is actually the projection into commonly-thought-of 'reality' of a self which cannot otherwise be on this journey? What if we are actually on some incredibly sophisticated Star Trek-like mission from somewhere else, and the thing we think of as our "body" is in truth an incredibly sophisticated spaceship designed and constructed to permit us to look around and actually participate here in this environment, where otherwise we could not survive? That our five senses are incredibly sophisticated instruments designed to detect certain kinds of emanations and waves which will allow us to fully interact with this place and with others of us who have arrived from "elsewhere," too.

Let's say that because these spaceships we inhabit are so sophisticated and complex, they do not hold together forever, even though they have a superbly engineered-in ability to repair themselves. The engineers and scientists back home have advised us that as of this stage, the generation ship we're using is not capable of repairing everything; for example, it cannot re-grow an external limb, or rapidly repair damaged internal communication strands, or information storage and computation tissue. And if the central circulating pump goes, all functions quickly cease. There is no backup. We'll be quickly popped back into our original reality –

home, as it were, "out of the game." But in every time some of us have come here to continue working on improvements.

Now let's imagine that the "I" of us is actually Captain James T. Kirk, sitting on the bridge somewhere inside, and, as any good captain, he receives only the distillations and summaries of the myriad of the ship's functions, perceptions and inputs. That while much of the ship's systems function automatically and without direct input from the Captain (each system commanded, of course, by a Scotty here and a Doc there), as long as things are running smoothly, he doesn't hear much from "below" other than run-of-the-mill status reports. Only when a problem arises is the Captain alerted.

The Captain can, of course, become involved in a more detailed basis with any of the functions of the ship, and he may from time to time visit the various areas of the ship to talk to the crew, listen to their suggestions and beefs, understand their problems and generally encourage morale.

Well, there is where our analogy breaks down, isn't it? In our human spaceship, the captain doesn't do that. No visits are ever made to the stalwart crew that runs the kneecap, or that mans the liver, spleen and pancreas, or precisely coordinates those 26 bones in our foot – not to mention the 100+ muscles – so the body can make it into the kitchen for another beer.

In all these years I'll be you've never even left your exalted perch behind the big windows to slide down your medulla oblongata and say hello to the tireless workers whose job it is to hold your head erect.

It's time to change that. Let's look at what to do. We'll learn "how" later.

It's All Play

The process begins and ends with letting go. First, letting go of our narrow concept of reality and becoming like little children again, believing that something everyone tells you is impossible can still be done. It's easier if you don't already believe it's impossible. When I took my 12-year-old son to Jack Houck's 348th PK Party, who was the first of the 30 people in the room to bend the bowl of a tablespoon in half? You guessed it. Children know the way, without anyone ever telling them. Step one is to become like a child.

It's *all* play, not work. In all of the magical processes of life, from silly spoon bending to faith healing to helping an athlete go that extra distance to win a gold medal, there are a few constants. First there is the attitude of joy, of play, of freedom.

Play Permits Creative Focus

Second we must absolutely focus on the desired result, shutting out everything else but the goal at hand, and creating the image of it <u>already being reality</u>. Don't "do it till it hurts," do it in a relaxed, playful state. If your knee hurts and you want to relieve the pain and heal the knee, teasing it and playing with it is better than getting intense and forceful. You know that fact if you've had children. If you want help, focus on the Light, the energy and power of God, whatever you imagine that to be, and imagine moving that energy into your knee, *and watch as it begins to reshape the cells, ligaments, tendons, etc., to perfect health.* It is not enough just to "send some healing energy down there." That may work, but in my experience it's both inefficient and insufficient. *To make it really work, tell it what you're doing. Talk to it, like it's your friend. Out loud.*

Remember, there's nothing mystical about this! We just don't understand yet how it works. And we don't even have to. That doesn't make it eerie, or sacred, or occult, it just makes it something on our platter of things to learn about in the future. Jeez!, only a couple hundred years ago we used to talk reverently, fearfully, beseechingly to the rain gods about rain. Not that long ago we burned people as sacrifices to make our lives go well. We're getting better, but we've got a long way to go still.

I took an early morning motivational course a few decades ago designed to help people change their careers, life directions, etc., by changing the way they looked at what was possible in their lives. The first morning we arrived (by 6:00AM by God! or they locked the doors on you) the leader had written on the blackboard "Congratulations, you have just successfully completed this course. Now all there is left to do is do it." Think about that for a moment, and you'll understand the meaning of this part of the process. Focus on the outcome, see it already done. Remember, don't worry about how. That's God's/ the Universe's / the Infinite's job.

The Captain Speaks (softly)

Now talk to your body. I always begin by giving it a little TLC, because God knows I don't get around my body the way I should. Sometimes the crew in an area is almost in mutiny before I pay attention and go for a visit.

And I don't go down there all highhanded, either; I go hat in hand to listen and help. Oh, yeah, in the beginning I once went to an aching knee and said, "Hey, what's the matter with you, get back to work! Stop hurting right now!" and I quickly got an earful and was in pain for several days more: *"Hey so-called Captain, foist of all, youse don't even come down heah ta check on us 'til we're screaming our bloody heads off, den youse storms in like some Nazi and tells us we're not doin' our frikkin' job! What makes ya t'ink you're ever gonna get anyt'ing out of us like dat, ya idjit?"* (I did notice some of them hiding what looked like union cards as I arrived.)

So, a little TLC is a good way to start. A few hugs around, some verbally expressed appreciation for the years of excellent service, then "What can I do to help?" And finally, invoking the power of healing: Remind them that they're fine, they have just been shaken up a bit, or ignored, or not fed well, etc., and you're going to change that right now. The Word from the Captain is "everything's okay now."

You know the attitude police adopt when they're about to arrest you? (Okay, you've never been arrested, but this is it anyway.) It's called "command authority," and it's taught in every police academy. When they turn that intense bearing on you, it's like a big beam of light is hitting you in the face. They can be as polite as a kindergarten teacher, but when they ask you to "step over here and take out your drivers license, please," if you're not an idiot you know that's what you're going to do.

That is the attitude of the Captain of your ship. The absolute surety that when you tell your cells that they're okay, and they're now going to return to doing their job perfectly, that's what they're going to do. When you tell your muscle it's not pulled, that it just got scared and it's fine now, that's the attitude with which you do it. Not a demand, but rather an *absolute knowingness* delivered with the power of the Light you have brought to the new image, resolving the confusion the cell or muscle had because of whatever trauma occurred. You speak with the full knowledge that the change is accomplished now, swiftly, and completely.

When the Captain instructs her crew to perform a task, she does not doubt that it will be carried out, she already knows it's done.

Everyday is Thanksgiving

The final step is giving thanks – to God, the universe, the Great Spirit, Allah, Krishna, whomever you envision the Maker of All to be, for the creation that has now occurred. Here's the trick: you do this *in spite of no physical evidence*, for the physical manifestation of a change in reality takes awhile (for "Lucy" and those of us who still believe in Time). And you're done.

Release and Forget It

At this point you are completely immersed into the new reality, all thought of what else was or might have been is gone.

The Captain does not wait and ask if the order has been carried out, he continues about his business knowing that it is done. And those are the words I like to use, "It is done."

I often see the "release" like a flock of birds I send out into the Universe to carry the message of the new reality to the "future," where it will manifest.

Don't sit there and wonder if it really worked, get up and go about your business. To paraphrase that message on the blackboard:

Congratulations, your healing has just successfully occurred. Now all there is left to do is forget about it and go play.

In the beginning, don't be surprised if it wears off. What happens is, that monster, fear, creeps back in. Like Freddie Kruger in the *Nightmare on Elm Street* movies, old monsters take a long time to die. Don't worry, if your confidence wanes, *do it again*.

Yes, the entire process. Especially the release at the end. If you walk away holding tight to the intention, the emotion, or your fear, shake it off. Wait awhile, and repeat.

Some Things to Do Along the Way

While you're playing this wonderful game, remember always that there is nothing "wrong' with anything you do. There's no judge, no someone out there watching you who afterward is going to analyze what you did and how you did it, no "way" that works or doesn't work. *The correct path is the one you take*, haltingly at first, perhaps (mine was), but at least you can explore freely, secure in the knowledge that when you're done, only you will know how it went. You won't get a report card or a periodic assessment from anyone but yourself. So…drop some old habits:

Touch Your Body!

Somewhere in our need to be "nice" many of us have forgotten that touching is more powerful than not touching. Oh, yes, over the past several decades healers have demonstrated how well they can pass healing energy to someone by putting their hands a couple inches above their body and visualizing the energy flowing between them. Massaging the aura, if you will.

If that works so well, imagine how much more efficient an energy transfer you get by actually *touching* the person! We're so afraid to make physical contact, even with ourselves! If there's a boil or a wound or a tumor in your body, and you can feel it, go after it! Touch it lovingly, massage it tenderly, get acquainted with it, inside and out. A good start is: "Hello friend, sorry I was afraid of you there for awhile! Let's get acquainted!"

But figuring these things out is only half the solution. Putting them into action every day is the other half. Oh well, something else to play with as you're beginning this wonderful game.

Touch your body while you talk to it, especially the area you're working on. Some of us have become so uncomfortable with ourselves that we're often even afraid to inspect a damaged or diseased part of us. C'mon, it's all US, it's not Me vs. My Body.

"Eeeww, that's awful, I don't even want to look at it" doesn't get us anywhere. How do you think a child feels if an adult – its parent – says, "Eeeww, you're just too ugly to look at"? That's what you're doing.

The skin wants attention just as much as any of the rest of us. Certainly infections and cuts need cleaning and mothering. I don't' care if you're a dad, mother it! And that pimple on your nose? Smile, and love it away. Oh, I know, it's so ugly even its mother wouldn't love it. But you ARE its mother, and you'd better, or it's going to sit there and whine at you from now until kingdom come! You've never heard a pimple whine? It sounds like this, "I can't believe my face is so broken out…" (It throws its voice.)

Take note: The old healing services weren't called "holding the hands close to the subject and praying," they were called "laying on of hands." Get to it.

"Don't Muss My Hair!"

"You can heal me, but don't muss my hair." Reminds me of the new Christian who wants to be baptized but doesn't want to get her hair wet by that sprinkly thing. I have no sympathy for you. In the church of my childhood we did full immersion – the dunk tank, us kids called it.

Well, sorry, this technique may just get your hair messed up…and your clothes, too. You might find yourself so involved with healing your body you wind up rolling on the floor in your room. I try to do it while I'm running, but different healers use different techniques. There's a wonderful process called "Transformational Breathing" which, when I did it one night at the Optimum Health Institute[16] in San Diego, it had me (and 20 others) writhing on the floor in an amazing, vibrant, religious experience, no drugs involved. Reminded me of my days in the Pentecostal church. We weren't called "holy rollers" for nothing.

If you've never meditated before, you may want to wait until you finish the book before starting to try the process. A more detailed description of how to do it is in Chapter XI and also in the Appendix.

When you do this, go deep inside, lose yourself in the experience. The more real it feels the better it works. Then go directly to the problem and start the dialogue. Whatever comes up is exactly right. As the Silva teachers said, and remote viewers

---

[16] See Chapter XIII

everywhere know, there's no wrong way, you're making it up anyway.

Don't edit what comes up, let your dialogue be as inane as it wants to be. Look at mine. After all these years, the Mental Normalcy Police haven't knocked on my door yet. Most important, enjoy it. You'll be amazed, surprised, overwhelmed. You'll laugh, and maybe cry. You'll feel a lot better afterward.

And who knows, you might even heal something!

◊

Casual Magic

One evening I was telling my friend Anna Stookey, at the time a massage therapist, about this concept, and when she heard what I was up to, her eyes opened wide and she exclaimed, "I've done that!" And then she proceeded to relate an experience she had with a therapy client who was about to undergo chemotherapy for cancer. He was troubled that the chemo would have all sorts of bad side effects, and wished he could do something to ameliorate them.

She suggested that as she worked on his body, they talk to it, and they did. She guided him to imagine himself inside his body, talking to his cells and explaining that this chemo was actually something good, something that he was looking forward to having done in order to help the body, and the cells shouldn't be afraid of it, because he actually wanted it. Anna says they went through this process for quite some time, and then the next day he went in for his first chemo treatment.

You already know what happened. Nothing. He didn't get sick, he didn't lose his hair, and the chemotherapy eradicated the cancer without any of the side effects that are normally expected.

The unexpected thing was that the lack of side effects scared his doctors! Their first reaction was that they hadn't given him enough of the drugs! They couldn't believe it. This was the first time that these experienced oncologists had ever *seen someone have no negative reaction to a regimen of chemotherapy.*

When I asked Anna what had made her think of this in the first place, she said it was because when she was in her mid-20s, she had had braces put on her teeth.

"My teeth hurt terribly for the first couple days," she said, "and even the pain medication they gave me didn't help. I needed to do something to relieve the agony, so it occurred to me that maybe my teeth were signaling pain because they were trying to alert me that something was wrong. That's what pain is for, after all. So I decided to tell them that while I appreciated their letting me know something was wrong, nothing actually was wrong, in fact I wanted the braces, and everything was all right.

"The pain stopped almost immediately."

Chapter VIII: Into the Depths of Fear

This one's tough. Remember the disclaimer at the beginning of this book. I do not recommend you try this yourself. Standard medical procedure is much the more logical, prudent path. Whatever you decide, you must take full responsibility for your actions. But here's what I did.

It's one thing to chat up your achy arm and leg muscles, or relax an organ that on any medical exam would show to be working normally, or even help your body tolerate real or anticipated pain. It's quite another to get it on with that part of your ship that holds your very life in its hands…your heart.

No one ever told you your heart was your friend. It's an organ that, sadly, we expect to "run down," to deteriorate over time. So many of us think of our bodies like we do our cars. "Well, after awhile it just falls apart!" That's a convenient image, but it leads us into bad places. We are not like our cars. I ask you, what car ever knitted a broken axle back together, or reconnected its own wiring? Not yet, anyway.

Experts tell us to eat right, exercise, and not to stress, for fear (fear!) that these things will cause our heart to fail us. But these are experts who only observe the heart from the outside, and they too often make assumptions that something is not possible just because no one has ever done it before. No nutritional expert I know of ever sat down and directly *asked* a heart what it really needs. And no heart surgeon I know of has ever suggested we have a little chat with that part of us which ought to be our best friend.

Along about the time I turned 50, I started having occasional chest pains. I had been a moderate runner for nearly 20 years and was in excellent health. But the pains kept coming – more ache than pain, really, but some minor tingling in my left arm and hand made my fear work overtime and then, of course, the sweating began. Real, or hypochondria? My first instinct was to go for a treadmill test, and its EKG showed frequent "PVC's" – pre-ventricular contractions – but the cardiologist said that wasn't necessarily unusual. Yeah, but they hurt. He concluded that "we should run some more tests," delicately leaving out the word *invasive*. I told him I'd *think* about it. Thoughts...

One Sunday, when I was feeling particularly achy in the left side of my chest, and felt my elbow and fingers tingle, I couldn't think of anything but "heart attack." I knew that modern medicine, like a caring father, would have picked me up and hauled me off to the hospital, but I had something else in mind – a treadmill test of my own. Refusing to be a victim of my own fears, and with the experience of my spider-web eye as background, I went to the gym, got on the treadmill, and started walking. At first I was terrified, but determined. What if I was wrong?

But I had decided I'd rather die acting on my beliefs than survive only because I was afraid of testing them.

On the treadmill I quickly put myself into the deepest meditative state I could reach. I floated my mind down to my heart and for the next 45 minutes we had a deep 'heart to heart' talk. I pulled no punches. I told my heart that I was scared to death. That I loved it and had tried for years to make sure it was strong and healthy, ever since my father's early heart attack had frightened me into a more or less healthy lifestyle.

I told it how much it meant to me and that whatever it needed me to do, I would be there and do it. I seemed to hear it say "clean it out," so I moved around to the various veins and arteries I imagined feeding into and out of it and shrunk myself down some more, so I could get into them. Then I conjured up a large bristle-brush, some imaginary "cleaning solution," and went to work. Outside my head, the strong beat of rock music was pounding in the room, and I was walking hard on the treadmill. Inside my head I was scrubbing those veins and arteries for all I was worth. I was inside my heart, brushing and scraping and cleaning to the beat of the music.

The intensity of the music increased, and the intensity of my treading went with it. I was holding on for dear life, working every muscle in my body in rhythm to the music, working away at those arteries inside my chest. I was the expert cleaning guy here to make those pathways shine like new again. I wasn't going to stop until every bit of crud and debris was completely gone. I worked as if my life depended on it. And I talked to each vein and artery, telling them just how clean they were getting, how perfect they were becoming once again. I might as well have been making love to my heart, that's how intense this relationship got.

After about 20 minutes of this, I began to notice that the pain in my chest was gone. My fear was gone, too, replaced by a powerful knowledge that I was changing things. I kept working. I knew my heart was going to be perfect when I was through, and I knew it had been asking for some serious attention from me.

After 30 minutes, my heart and I began to relax, we knew that everything was all right. Now it was as if we were dancing together. It seemed to almost snuggle up against me in happiness. I imagined I could feel the free flow of blood and energy through it, the ease of contraction and release of its beats. The music was still pounding, I was still working hard on the treadmill, but tears of release and relief started down my face, tears of love for my wonderful heart.

I stayed there, inside my heart, for another ten minutes or so, enjoying the feeling that all was well. I was running now, and feeling perfect. Then I slowly lowered the speed of the machine, and started becoming aware of my surroundings again. I thanked my heart from the bottom of my…self…and told it I would never forget to show it my love and appreciation ever again.

It was all over in 45 minutes. Half an hour later I was home, trying to tell my wife what had happened. I have never had a chest pain or PVC since.

I love my heart. And I talk to it often.

Open Your Heart

Recently a news report came out describing how scientists have concluded that the brain is not the only "brain" in our body; that, in fact, the heart is as much of a brain as the brain itself when it comes to our emotional life! Well knock me over with a toothpick, isn't that just what folk traditions have been telling us forever!

The heart is the seat of our emotional being! How many poems and songs and ancient stories do we have to hear before we get it? Let's see…there's Valentine's Day…and "heartfelt thanks," and "speaking from the heart," and "my heart's desire," and "you gotta have heart," and "What does your heart tell you?" and, the big one, "Love." Fill in the blank: Love comes from the _____. (You didn't write brain, did you?)

And it takes a scientific study to get us to pay attention! Classic, isn't it?

"Hard Hearts" and Hard Heads

As I mentioned, I'm a ham radio operator – a practitioner of that now dying art of communication via short-wave radio with other hams all over the world, including the late King Hussein of Jordan, the Sultan of Brunei, various Arab sheiks, the crew of the Space Shuttles, and US and Russian South Pole Station scientists. Part of the fun of this hobby is, you never know who you're going to be chatting with when you turn on the radio.

The other day I was listening on my radio, and I heard a fellow say that he had taken a radio he no longer used down to a local swap meet and tried to sell it for much less than it was worth.

No takers – at that price they suspected it was no good. Finally he put a sign on it reading, "FREE," and it was shunned even more. Everyone seemed to think there was a gimmick, after all no one would give a good radio away free.

Finally, he taped seven one-dollar bills onto it and enlarged the sign to "WORKING RADIO FREE. DON'T HAVE ROOM FOR IT, PLEASE TAKE."

No one touched it.

When your basic outlook on life is that someone's out to take advantage of you, you pass up a lot of wonderful opportunities. The underlying proposition of our culture seems to be that everyone's out to get us, and if we're not really careful, they will. Then people make millions convincing us we must buy security devices…or else. So we don't trust anyone except our friends, and even then we have to be ready, they might betray us at any time.

We even learn as kids, "Be Prepared." So we gird up, brace up and ride into the wild jungle, ready to pounce before we're pounced upon. We're so ready to defend ourselves that some have started carrying concealed weapons everywhere, like it's the Wild West of the 1850's, and we react to any sudden movement. Especially those unexpected movements made on the freeway by metal steeds ridden by strangers – each one a potential enemy.

But after years of being ever-prepared, we are no longer able to disarm. We become hypertensive, can't sleep, have trouble breathing, develop tension headaches and muscle aches, and even our organs begin to have trouble functioning. Most obvious is our heart, so long neglected and deprived of attention or ability to express itself, it literally attacks us.

"Heart Attack." What a fascinating, scary, two-word terror. The medical description, always in Latin, was *coronary thrombosis*: literally, "heart occlusion." Occlusion – stoppage. Not as in "ceasing to work," (yes, that, too) but as in the clogging of a pipe.

So we have a heart that is clogged up and can't pump. And then it attacks! "Attack of the Clogged Heart! – Now Playing." What's the line, "Use it or lose it."? An unused heart shrivels up and rusts away. What is arterial plaque around the heart but an organic version of rust and corrosion?

But if our assumption that "our bodies communicate with us" is to be useful, then clearly we must believe that the heart has to be trying to get our attention for a long time before it starts to attack us. Which brings up another question:

Why do more men die of heart attacks than women? I have an idea: we men think too much. We operate out of the brain, out of *reason*, out of an eons-old tradition of war, while women tend more to operate from their heart. The need for men to "gird for battle" has been around for so many millennia that it has become a part of our genes, while for just as long women have cared for the children and the home.

Girding for battle requires a steeling of one's being – holding tension, being prepared, staying focused, parrying with the competition, even killing. Caring for another requires being open and yielding, listening to their wants and needs, being in tune with nature. You sure can't kill when your heart's open.

From our traditions, then, women's hearts are open; men's are closed. So men experience heart attacks more often than women do…because women's hearts don't have to attack – they get the attention they need with just a little nudge.

I'm generalizing, now, but see if this doesn't just about fit: Women are accustomed to sensing when a child needs attention – a little TLC, some quiet time. Men typically never notice until the child makes a fuss or throws a tantrum, and then the man too often insists the mother deal with it.

So men, wake up! Take a page from your wife's book of life, and listen to your heart. I don't mean the physical muscle, I mean that Heart we all hear trying to get a word in edgewise every time we make a decision or a judgment. It's as simple as the ubiquitous freeway dialogue you hear every day: "Hey, jerk, you cut me off, you $^%#@!!!" That's your head talking, and your heart is cut off from the conversation. If you gave your heart the slightest input in the conversation, it might sound like this: "Hey, you scared me, but you know what?...I'm not going to judge why you did that or what's going on in your life, I just pass a little love on to you and hope all is well."

Sounds like something out of the hippy '60s, doesn't it? "Peace, brother." Well, do you want to get even with a stranger who you (mostly wrongly) perceive to have attacked you, or do you want to live a little longer, a lot happier? Hmmm: Get Even vs. Live Longer. Your choice. You might choose to get even. As for me, I'll just try to stay out of your way. *(NOTE TO SELF: Remember this when driving!)*

Judgment kills, too...us. Most of us go around judging everyone, especially people we don't know and therefore can't possibly know why they act the way they do. And in those times, when we act out of our head we're always wrong.

I remember sitting in church some time ago watching the people enter and sit down. We're a group of varied ethnic and cultural types, but any anthropologist worth his salt would quickly note that our dress and demeanor fit within certain stereotypical modern American parameters.

This particular Sunday a stranger entered, and he was strange in many obvious ways. From his heavy Doc Martin boots to his out-of-time clothes to his eccentric hair. Oh, his hair! It was cut in a perfect Mohawk – an *orange* Mohawk. A completely shaved head except for the two-inch stripe of rigidly vertical orange colored hair running from his forehead to the nape of his neck. It was clear to me that this fellow didn't belong among us. Add the kicker: he was black. Not too many black people in our services either, unfortunately. But nobody, black, white or green, with an orange Mohawk and Doc Martins, to be sure.

Nevertheless, as the service began, I closed my eyes and tried to forget he was there. I couldn't, of course. All through the service all I could think of was, "What are you doing here you weird person…have you come to deliberately disrupt this worship service? Who's going to tell this fellow he doesn't belong in this house of God. (Note that: "in this house of God!" – what egotist determines just who are children of God and who are not?!)[17]

A good hour into the service, when guests and visitors were being acknowledged, Stranger stood and began to speak. "Oh, no," I thought, "here it comes!"

"I am happy to be back with this wonderful fellowship," he began. "I have been traveling for more than two years, and I want to tell you some stories of my journey…" Whereupon he began to talk of having walked – walked! – across the United States in the past two years on *a mission of peace*. He talked of the time his leg was broken when he was struck by a car at night on the highway, and of how he and the driver became fast friends during his hospitalization. He talked of meeting families and children and caring people all over the country, who took him in, and fed him, and shared stories of their lives with him as he traveled. He talked softly, wisely, of the kindnesses of the people of America, and of the goodness he found wherever he traveled.

He had come to our service to bring us hope for the future of mankind, experienced firsthand on the highways and byways of our nation.

This strange, orange-haired fellow was the Peace Pilgrim, the fourth, actually, carrying on a tradition begun years ago of walking throughout the land sharing the joy of friendship, fellowship and peace among people everywhere. His words touched our hearts deeply, and we were profoundly moved by his life's devotion.

---

[17] See the judgmental attitude I finally had to deal with in the Epilogue.

For the rest of the service I sat quietly in my seat, feeling abject shame for my judgmental stupidity.

We know the correlation between judgment and the heart. The Bible says it clearly, "…and they hardened their hearts…" Any cardiologist will tell you, hard hearts don't work very well.

Open your heart, soften it. Let it be the place from which you speak, and it will be infinitely less disposed to attack you.

◊

Heart May Be Able to Mend Itself After Heart Attack

Therapy to Regenerate Heart Muscle Still Years Away, Experts Caution

By Neil Osterweil   June 6 -- Conventional medical wisdom takes another hit with news that heart muscle cells appear capable of re-growing after a heart attack, suggesting that it may be possible to coax the heart into repairing itself, report researchers in what's being hailed as a landmark study published in the June 7 issue of *The New England Journal of Medicine*.

(as reported on WebMD)

Chapter IX: Acting on Your Belief

It's one thing to try this magic on yourself. It's quite another to do it with someone else – especially a child, and especially when the injury might seem serious. Some would call me an irresponsible father for what I'm about to relate. All I know is that so far as I'm concerned, if I'm going to believe something, I must act on that belief, especially when it's tough, or else I should change my belief.

When my daughter Annie was eight, she and I were spending a Saturday morning in a local park, watching her older brother at Little League practice. Annie was playing on the rings in a jungle gym beside the ball field, staying happily occupied. She had been taking gymnastics for a couple years, and was quite agile on them, but still, the concerned father in me made me stand close, especially because these rings, unlike the ones at her gym, were fairly high – probably five feet off the ground, and there was nothing but hard ground beneath them.

She played on them for awhile, so clearly comfortable and adept that I must have dropped my guard slightly. Suddenly without warning, she fell. Time stopped, it was the classic slow-motion experience. I lunged, but even as close as I was, I could not react quickly enough to catch her. Within inches of my outreaching hands, she fell the five feet to the ground, landing squarely on her back and head with a sickening thud.

I knelt beside her immediately, in shock that I hadn't been able to catch her. As she lay there in that moment of silence that followed, I once again had two choices. The first was what I wanted to do: grab her, scream for someone to call 911, and then watch helplessly as she was whisked off to an emergency room where a team of pros would put her through tests and x-rays to determine if she had broken her back, or had a concussion.

The second choice was what I did. I took a deep breath and remembered that at this moment – the Schrödinger's cat moment – it was just as possible that she was perfectly fine, that the fall had just knocked the wind out of her, and in a few minutes she would be running around playing again, having all but forgotten the fall.

"Just as possible…" Physicists from Einstein to Hawking have told us that at any given moment, the future is not yet determined, that all possible futures still exist, no matter how small their likelihood, no matter what our fears tell us. I knew in my head that in the face of no evidence – even in the face of my own fear – it was possible that she was fine. The problem I faced in that moment was acting on that belief, wholly and completely, and quickly.

In that tiny moment of suspended time, while my precious little girl was still taking in what had happened and before she started to cry, I decided that this was the future I would give all of my attention – my intention – to: a future in which she was perfectly fine. If our actions and beliefs have any weight on what happens next, I was going to bet in that direction, even with the health of the little girl I loved with all my heart.

Some would say I was a foolish father; that my daughter's health was definitely not something to be gambling on like this. They caution that it's at times like these when you must fall back on the collective wisdom of the culture: don't move her, call an ambulance, let the experts handle it. You could do irreparable damage otherwise.

But I answer that if you set out to learn truth, and you learn something that with all your intellect and sense you believe must certainly be true, then when the moment arrives you must put that belief into action in your life. You cannot go on being the person you used to be, when you feel for sure that the new way is real. If you don't walk the talk, you're wasting your life.

And so I lay down beside my daughter on the dirt, and in that second before she could utter the first cry, I laughed. It wasn't a laugh that came easily, at first I had to force it through the fear welling up inside me. But I laughed anyway, and then gradually it became a real laugh. She looked at me, and I saw a faint smile creep onto her face. "I'll bet you scared yourself, didn't you?" I said. She nodded, "It hurts." And then came the question all parents must answer correctly: "Am I okay Daddy?"

I smiled at her, and with the lightness that comes with a good laugh, I said, "You're fine, honey," and then I started to improvise. In my best imitation of a Disney cartoon character, I said, "But you sure scared those poor cells in your back. I'll bet they don't know WHAT happened! One minute they're busy moving your muscles around like normal, and the next second, 'bang' – 'what was that?' they're yelling. Heeeeyyyyy! What're you doin' to us, anyway?"

And she started to laugh.

I remembered that cells, when traumatized or stressed, secrete lactose, which anyone who exercises experiences as that achy pain following a hard workout. Gathering my courage, I quickly added: "I'll bet those cells peed in their pants!" And she laughed harder.

"Let's go down there and talk to them, okay?" I said. She nodded, and I continued: "Okay, close your eyes, we're going to jump down your shoulders, and here we go, getting smaller and smaller, down your back, into those muscles…there they are… Hey, cells, sorry about that. Didn't mean to scare you! You're okay, though, just a little surprise, but you're fine. Now you tell them, honey." And in her own way she repeated what I had said.

I hadn't tried to move her yet, we just lay on the ground together and played this silly game. Then she asked, "How come it still hurts, Daddy?" I stayed on message: "Well, remember, those poor cells got so scared that they peed their pants, and what hurts is the cell pee you're feeling. We'll just have to tell your body to get rid of it, quick." She thought that was the funniest thing she'd ever heard, and laughed so hard she forgot to be afraid. "Cell pee. I feel the cell pee in my back!"

After a few minutes of laughing about this together, I casually asked her if she wanted to get up and brush herself off. She said yes, and I helped her sit up, then moved my hand along her spine, telling her I was going to help her body get rid of that cell pee. She laughed again. I was feeling for anything unusual, while silently sending her whatever healing energy I could imagine. Then I helped her to her feet, and held her hand as we slowly walked to the car a few yards away.

For the next half hour we sat in the back seat together, doors open, watching her brother play baseball and talking about cell pee and how to talk to your body when it thinks it's hurt. Then we talked about school, and other things. In another few minutes she was running around the park again, playing.

Next morning there was no residual aching when she woke up, and by the time she got to school, she had forgotten all about the fall, except to tell her friends about how cells pee their pants when they are surprised. I expect her friends think her daddy's crazy. Or, maybe this idea started getting around that very day.

I can imagine what would have happened had I made another choice. I certainly would have told her not to move, just as we're cautioned to do. For fifteen minutes, while someone frantically called the paramedics and they came, sirens blaring, she would have lain on the ground crying, mostly because she would have sensed the anxiety and fear in me and those who would have invariably gathered around her, looking down at her with serious adult concern on their faces. If an adult's afraid, there's certainly something a child has to fear.

Then the uniformed strangers would have arrived, and would have been especially careful as they lifted her onto a stretcher. They would have strapped her down just to be safe, and put her into a strange vehicle for the trip to the hospital, where even more strangers would have taken over, and with concerned precision, performed tests on her with cold steel utensils and detached professionalism. Their mouths would have spoken words of comfort, but she would have heard instead the concern in their voices.

Her mother would have arrived, face taut with fear, and Annie would have released her terror hysterically onto Mommy, who would have asked a hundred questions, and responded internally, if not externally, with her own anxiety that something might be seriously wrong with her little girl. Annie would have felt her mother's anxiety, and it would have scared her more.

Hours later, the trauma of the experience completely absorbed by the little girl, a diagnosis would have been delivered. It probably would have included words like "trauma" and "possible compression of a disk" and maybe "fracture" or "concussion," and end with "We should look at her again in a week or so and see how she's doing."

To the little girl who simply fell off the rings on the playground, this would have been an intensely terrifying experience, with long-lasting consequences, no matter the ultimate conclusion. She would have braced up, and tensed up, and whatever damage might have been done by the fall would have been multiplied in her mind and, exacerbated by her actions, would have resolved into days of a sore back and who knows what else.

I cannot tell you what you should do if a similar situation occurs in your life, I would be foolish to do so. But I can relate my own experiences, and hope that you can imagine some possibilities beyond reacting in terror, fear, and taking what too many lawyers and concerned bureaucrats call "safe and appropriate action."

Many psychologists these days tell us that the terror and fear of our experiences go straight into the parts of our body that are most traumatized at the moment…to stay forever. I conclude that had I taken the other path, my daughter might have had some kind of back problems or pain for years. In this case, however, the whole thing was completely forgotten, mentally and physically in a few days.

So two things were at work here: First, since the future truly was not there yet, and there was no "reality" in which existed damage to Annie's back (the only realities could have been in her mind or mine, at that point, assuming Einstein's conclusion that there is no objective reality, but only that which is experienced by the observers), it therefore was still quite possible that nothing was wrong with her – that all that had happened was that she got the "wind knocked out of her."

I believe that it was equally possible that she had received a debilitating injury to her spine, but given the choice, I chose to act in the direction of the best possibility. If our beliefs in any way affect the future, then I was determined to move Probability toward the way I wanted that future to be experienced.

Second, if I didn't quickly find a place within myself where I could truly believe that she was fine, she would sense it, and whatever inner workings were under the direction of her own thought processes would turn negative, too. If my belief structure affects the outcome of an experience, then hers certainly would, too, and I had to make sure she had no thought of anything being wrong.

Thus I accepted the great challenge offered by Dr. Norman Cousins[18]: in the midst of the worst adversity, laugh.

◊

---

[18] Former editor of *The Saturday Review*, professor at Washington University, St. Louis, healed himself from a debilitating illness with vitamin C and laughter, detailed in his book *Anatomy Of An Illness*.

"...in many incarnations of the idea there are ultimately infinite universes. This would also include other copies of ourselves."

- From an interview with Columbia University Physicist Brian Greene in Newsweek's "There May Be Infinite Universes — and Infinite Versions of You"

- by Douglas Main, Newsweek July 9, 2015

Chapter X: Look What You Did to Me!

Remember the first step I told you about? The letting go part? That's the hardest part.

One of the things children do when you ask them to say, "Not a word of truth to it," after an injury is say, "NO!" And then continue crying and holding the hurt part of their body. That is in fact what all of us tend to do. There seems to be something in our makeup that wants to feel the hurt, or at least we are afraid to let it go, for fear it will hurt more when we do.

It is a difficult thing to let go of a banged toe, relax it, and tell it that it's fine, when all our instincts urge us to grab it and tense up our entire body with the pain. But it is the fastest way to healing.

When some small injury has occurred and my kids don't want to "play the game," I say, "So you just want to feel the pain and not make it better?" And they say, "Yes!" So I laugh. Which sometimes makes them laugh, and sometimes makes them mad at me. And then I try again. When they're hurt, just as with Annie on the playground, I sit down with my children and tell them how everything's okay, and coax them gently to let go and allow the possibility (I don't use that word) that everything is okay. Gradually, they do. Most of the time.

But some of the time they – and we – want to hang on to the pain, often just for spite, just as often for attention. Who among us doesn't like having the world screech to a halt on our behalf? In recent years, out-of-work or well-meaning lawyers frequently take advantage of that human inclination, and in so doing, greatly magnify our problems (in both meanings of that phrase).

Added to the attention getting hurt attracts to us, we have this attitude that if someone hurts us they should be punished for it, and how better to punish them than to wear a big bruise, be in serious pain, and have everyone feel sorry for us – and of course see them angry on our behalf at the person who hurt us.

The best example is a minor car accident, where the driver who's clearly not at fault limps out of the car holding their back or neck, and complains of whiplash. Even if they have whiplash, the incentive to really be hurt, either in order to show the bastard who hit them what a jerk he is or to collect a big check somewhere down the line, is going to make their pain worse, because at that moment there is not much incentive to be okay.

If you were playing touch football in your own back yard and your son hit you from behind and it gave you the same injury, you'd think long and hard before spending too much of your next six months in the doctor's office, wouldn't you? But when somebody says, "You can collect thousands if you start spending lots of time in physical therapy," there's incentive to not walk away and say, "I'm fine." At times like that, it's pretty hard to convince yourself you're really okay.

The only problem is, when you decide to be hurt, you intensify the pain, and so have to carry it around with you for weeks, maybe even months, instead of quickly getting rid of it. You may have to spend lots of time with extremely cooperative doctors and physical therapists working on something that you didn't need to fix in the first place. After all, every hour you spend with them is an hour more of fee they get from the insurance company, so where's *their* incentive to pronounce you well?

But then there's the issue of self respect…but hey, where money's involved what's a little stretching of the truth? It wasn't MY fault, HE did it, and HE SHOULD PAY! All the while forgetting that you're paying just as big a price as the poor guy who hit you. So, instead of honest, self-respecting healthy people who get into accidents once in awhile and shrug them off, we have become a culture of blamers and suers, with a cadre of doctors and therapists who don't mind a bit helping us rehabilitate – for pay.

It's hard to heal yourself if there's something that causes you, consciously or sub-consciously, to not want to be healed. The way we react to pain and injury is devious. I recently read about a therapist who worked mainly with obese people. As he helped them deal with a particular issue in their lives, they would lose weight – 20 pounds or so – and stabilize again at the reduced weight.

Each time another deep-seated issue was resolved in therapy, their weight would go down another step, until the point when they were dealing with something they could not, or did not want to, face. At that point their weight loss stopped. No matter what diet they went on, if they couldn't deal with the psychological issue they were stuck on, their weight would eventually return to that level.

One autumn I chaperoned my son's sixth-grade class on an overnight camping trip in the local mountains; I was one of a handful of dads and moms recruited to help with driving and tents and cooking and mostly just standing around looking appropriately adult so the kids wouldn't get too out of hand.

This group of 25 boys and girls runs the classic American gamut of skinny Taylor Swift wanna-be girls to the too-many-Twinkies boy who hasn't yet realized he can run and play. In the language of one parent, he's a "choleric-melancholic," or, in everyday words, life's terrible and he complains about everything.

On the second day of the camp out, Too-Many-Twinkies (TMT, let's call him) was hurrying down a hillside trying to keep up with the other boys when he tripped, fell, and rolled a few feet before coming to a stop on a flat trail. The other kids ran for help. I was the nearest adult they could find, but I was certainly not what he was expecting.

With how he was moaning and groaning, I'm sure that some other parent might have helped him to the car and driven him to the hospital for an MRI. He was already talking about X-rays when I arrived at the scene, and I laughed. That really pissed him off. "I'm hurt, don't you understand!?" he screamed, continuing to moan between breaths. "My shoulder...my leg...I have to go to the hospital!"

But he was standing up, and when I brushed the grass off him he didn't wince. It seemed like maybe he'd never fallen down a hill before – a sad statement to make about any kid who's 11 years old. Anyway, I hugged him, and in between his moans I told him to repeat after me, "I'm fine! It was fun rolling down the hill."

He wouldn't. "I'm NOT fine!!" he demanded. "I *knew* I shouldn't have come on this trip, I told my parents not to send me! And see what happens!?"

I laughed again. "Yes you are fine! Just imagine you were playing a game, and you rolled down the hill for fun! You'd be laughing now."

"Yeah? What if YOU rolled down the hill," he retorted, "YOU wouldn't be laughing!"

"Oh yes I would. In fact, come on, we'll go back up there and roll down together. Let's go!" I took his hand and tried to walk up the hill with him, but he wouldn't come. Something about this 50-year-old man daring him to roll down the hill with him stopped him for just the moment I needed. "Oh, so you WANT to feel bad, huh?" I chided. "Okay, you can either do what I tell you and feel better, or you can go on feeling bad, it's your choice."

Not surprisingly, he said, "Yes, I want to feel bad!" I laughed again and started to walk away. "Okay, then, go on, go feel bad, I can't help you. But if you change your mind, let me know, and we'll take the pain away. It's magic." I said.

He walked away a few feet, and I stood there. Then he turned around and walked back to me, glaring at me, saying nothing. I smiled, and took his head in my hands. "I know some magic," I said, and I'm going to teach it to you. You know that aching in your shoulder and leg you feel?"

"Yes," he replied grumpily.

"Let's take it away, shall we?"

"Okay."

"Say this: 'There's not a word of truth to it.'"

"What good is that?"

"It's part of the magic."

Hesitation, then he mumbles almost unintelligibly: "Nod-a-wort-uh-tru-tot."

"Good, say it again so your body can hear you."

Barely audible: "Nod-a-word-uh-tru-tuit"

"Did the fall hurt your mouth?"

"No."

"So say it like you actually believe it, then."

"I don't believe it."

"Then we can't work the magic. You have to ACT like you believe it. See, your muscles got scared when they hit the ground hard like that, because they're not used to doing that, so you've got to tell them they're okay. If you were in a football game it'd be okay, wouldn't it?"

"Yes."

"Then just tell them they're as okay as they would have been if you had been rolling around for fun in a football game."

"Okay."

"Out loud."

"Okay." Hesitation. "There's not a word of truth to it."

"What do you mean when you say that?" I asked.

"That they're okay."

"Tell them that."

More hesitation, but getting into it, now. "Hey muscles, you're okay."

"Tell them you love them."

He looked at me funny.

"Laugh at them, then, and tell them they're really fine."

He fakes a little laugh, and says, "Hey muscles, you're really fine."

I hugged him again, and said, "How do you feel now? Still hurt?"

"A little."

"Still want to go to the hospital?"

"No, I want to catch up with Tommy and the guys."

"That's the magic I was talking about. Now you can use it anytime you think you might be hurt."

He runs off. RUNS off! To join the others.

For awhile I watched him play with the other kids, completely forgetting that he'd ever fallen. At lunch, an hour or so later, the class and parents, probably 30 of us in all, joined hands in a large circle before eating. TMT came running into the eating area, late as usual, and had to break the line somewhere to join in. He walked around the circle until he came to me, and broke in to hold my hand. That was all the acknowledgement I ever got...or ever needed.

You have to want to be healed, to be healed.

◊

"...all life is interconnected and interdependent...we are part of a matrix of life...spacetime itself arises from consciousness, not consciousness from spacetime."

- Stephan A. Schwartz
"The 8 Laws of Change," Park Street Press
by permission of the author

Chapter XI: Finding Your Own Path

Ever have one of those days when you feel just a little down? There doesn't seem to be a reason to get out of bed, and when you do, nothing seems to go right. So you eat something really junky, like a donut or two, to feel a bit perkier, follow it with some intense caffeine, and that works for about an hour, and then the crash comes, and you feel worse, plus you're now frustrated that you ate the donuts. You just feel like sitting around feeling sorry for yourself, so you do.

That's when you turn on the TV for a distraction, and even then you get barraged with news on the latest serial killing or the Palestinians and Israelis fighting again or some outlaw group in Lower Slobbovia stealing a shoulder-fired atomic weapon, and all your favorite characters on TV are getting divorced or cancer or die on the operating table, and every talk show is about politics or has stories on beauty queens who gut pigs for fun or men who have fewer than six toes…and show you. In the immortal words of the old vaudeville routine, "Is that what's getting you down, Bunky?"

Well, life always presents us opportunities, doesn't it? Turn off the TV, close your computer, put your iPhone in the freezer, put out the cat, or put the cat in the freezer and your iPhone outside, and find a chair in your favorite room that's not facing a screen of any kind except the one that gives you a gander at the trees. Or sit on the floor. Or go sit on the porch. Get somewhere you're not used to being, and sit down. Stay there doing nothing for two whole minutes. Two minutes. Hard, isn't it? No noise, no distractions, only the incessant chatter of the mind. We really go out of our way not to do this these days. We don't even drive in our cars anymore without talking on the phone and listening to the radio at the same time.

I read recently that teenage skateboarders think of getting hurt as a good thing. They consider it a way of feeling something. As if it takes actual pain to cut through the numbness they have generated for themselves already by age 15. Thousand of hours of brain-numbing television, social media and 20,000 commercials a year will do that to you.

So two minutes of silence for most of us is terrifying. Wanna see your addictions up close and personal? Sit there for five minutes, doing nothing. Nothing but thinking. Apparently this generation took Grandma's "Devil makes work for idle hands" adage way too much to heart.

Sense Your Body

While you're sitting there, instead of trying to keep your hands off a keyboard or remote, spend fifteen seconds sensing your body. Go inside, as you will see in the next pages, and just feel it. You know how a cold comes on, don't you? It creeps up on you. First you feel a little sneeze that's different than your normal ones, or you feel a slightly swollen place in your nose. If it's going to be an infection, maybe one side of your mouth is tender, along the gum line. And you know that in two days it's going to be in the back of your throat, and in two more you're going to be down with some kind of bronchitis or strep throat and green stuff will be coming out of your nose.

We don't just wake up with this stuff, we get ample warning. But most of us aren't paying attention – and if we are, we don't think there's anything we can do about it anyway, so we just grit our teeth and block it out. We can usually feel a cold coming on, and ills in the rest of our body announce themselves, too.

But now you have a plan. Once you've been told by your body, in its quiet way, where the problem is, GO THERE AND FIX IT! At least have a loving, caring conversation with wherever the problem is. Give it 20 minutes – TWENTY MINUTES - of actual attention and dialogue. It sounds like an eternity, but it's less than the length of a sit-com and there are no commercials. Plus, I promise you, once you're in, the time will fly by.

During that time, be with whatever muscle or tissue or organ or pain that's getting your attention. Do all the things this book talks about – all the things you would do to a child who came to you in need of comfort.

And then you can take your favorite medicines and drugs if you want. No Army ever travels with just one weapon. But sometimes if PsyOps[19] and diplomats do their job really well, those big weapons that blow up things are never needed.

Once again (by now it should be painless and simple), this is the easiest part. Doing it is the hardest.

The Steps to Learning to Talk to Your Body (The Long Way)

There are as many paths to awareness in the blank period as there are people. Here is one way to find your way in. However you do it, once you're there, wander around a bit, like a child at the beach. Grownups are too often content to find a place in the sand, sit down and veg. Kids like to wander around and see what's there. They pick up driftwood and seaweed, dig in the sand, kick over mussels and shells.

If you've never done anything like this before, pick someplace where you don't normally do anything else even remotely similar, because some old habit will compete for your attention – like the couple that can't make love in their bed because they keep falling asleep, but have no trouble in the guest bedroom.

If you meditate already, and you "move toward the light" during the process, try something different this time. Once you're settled, wander around a bit -- take an exploratory walk in the space. Better, make it a hop, skip and jump. See what you find there – you might be surprised what the light illuminates. From this place you can go anywhere, just decide where you want to

---

[19] Psychological Operations, the strategic military unit designed to mold public opinion

visit and take off. If you're afraid or unsure, take the light with you. Better to see by, anyway.

No matter what, don't take this whole trip seriously, and don't be afraid when you get down there, like you're entering a forbidden area or something. Too many people have convinced us there is something scary there, or, just as bad, something we must be reverent in the face of. The "light" must be God, and we must approach it in reverent awe. Nothing could be further from the truth. The light is just bright because we've been in the dark forest for so long. Now we can finally see. And what there is to see is fun, playful, and filled with joy. Because it is creation, whatever we want to create becomes real, there in our mind.

There is no wrong way to play this game.

Step I: First Relax

You are the Captain, be not afraid.

Find a private place to sit or lie down where you can stay for some length of time without becoming uncomfortable. You can even do it while running or walking, if it won't bother you knowing that there might be other people listening to you. I like to get the blood circulating because I feel like the more oxygen getting to my brain while I'm doing this the better. However you relax, relax, and close your eyes.

Now we're going to move into that blank period of our reality. Remember, like a child. It should be a fun imaginary experience, but at first it may be a little disorienting, or even scary. Don't worry, you're never alone. You're imagining everything you think and do, and it's all under your direct control at all times. If it becomes too much, just stop, open your eyes, and go get a beer or something. This should be fun, stay light. (Maybe a *light* beer?)

Step 2: Explore, Create, Imagine

If you know how to meditate, start that process, and go into the place where you normally go. If you typically go "to the light," stop before you begin that, and skip on to Step 2A, below.

If you aren't accustomed to meditating, get very comfortable, close your eyes, toss away your inhibitions and crank up your imagination. After you're comfortable and relaxed, close your eyes and imagine you've drifted into an empty, dark space. You look around and see that you're actually in space, there are stars all around you, and you can see the circles of the paths of the planets. Everything is moving slowly, as in a slow and graceful dance. As you watch this "dance of the spheres," you begin to see in the distance an object moving toward you. As it approaches, slowly and gracefully, turning slowly on itself, you see that it is the number 3.

As you watch the 3 glide closer to you, notice all the detail about it. See if the sides are smooth or rough, shiny or dull, metal, wood, plastic, whatever they are, notice it, as it moves toward you. Then notice that it is three-dimensional, and look at the way the number is formed. Is it hollow, like this 3, or is it fat like this **3**? Maybe it's angular, like this 3. However it appears, take a thorough look at it.

Look at the sides, and see how the pieces are joined together. Maybe this is the work of a lone carver, or maybe it is has been extruded from a mold. Maybe it's nickel, or titanium, or stainless steel that has been welded together. Or maybe it's made out of leaves and grass, like a thatched roof. Whatever you see, see it clearly, and in great detail.

As it moves quite close to you now, you will see that it is very big, much bigger than you are, and that it has a hole through it easily big enough for you to glide through. Also, you can make yourself smaller if you like, and swim through the hole in the 3 as if you're gliding underwater through a beautiful cave. Notice as you go what the inside of the hole looks like, and then flip your fins and cruise on out the other side, into the beautiful blackness of space once again.

Enjoy the view of the stars and the rings of the planets' paths, maybe you'll see a few shooting stars while you're there, but then notice in the distance another objecting moving toward you. As it draws near, you see it is the number 2, just like the 3 before. As it approaches, notice all the detail about it. See what shape of 2 it is, perhaps this one: **2**, this one: *2*, or this one: **2**, or even this one: **2**. Like the 3, it can be as simple or ornate as you imagine.

Now as the 2 moves close to you, and you see how large it is, notice that there is a hole in its side, too. As with the 3, glide through the hole, and out the other side into space once again. Enjoy the comfortable trip.

Now in the distance is the 1, moving slowly toward you. Observe it as you have the others, then as it nears, notice a hole in the center of it and glide through it out to the other side.

Now you will see a formless place, an opening to somewhere else. The shape of the opening is the number 0, and you are moving toward it slowly and gracefully. As you approach the 0, move through its center and descend slowly down into an elevator, your personal elevator, which has been waiting for you. Look at the elevator in detail. Is it a small French style elevator, with wrought iron filigree everywhere, or is it a sleek elevator found in modern office buildings? Or maybe it's an industrial elevator, with a rope to close the double doors. Whatever you see, that's your elevator.

Close the doors, if that's necessary, and then notice on the side wall the number 9. The elevator will begin to descend under your control, from 9 to 8 and so on down to 1. As it does, be sure to clearly see the numbers as they go by. If you can't, slow down the elevator until you do see the number, then descend to the next number, until you reach 1.

Step 2A. The elevator will stop at 1. Step or float out, and you will find yourself in a room with hallways leading in various directions. Look around, see how it's laid out and decorated. Take a look at a few of the hallways, but don't go down any of them yet.

This is your launching center. From here you can travel to any part of your body at will. Each hallway is actually a nerve pathway which will lead you to whatever area of your body you want to go to. One leads to the heart and lungs, another out the shoulders, down the arms and into the tips of each finger. Another pathway will take you to the abdomen, or genitals, or down your legs to your knees and feet.

There's a pathway from here to every point in your body, and you never get lost. All you have to do is decide that the hallway on your left, for example, leads you down your spinal cord to the back of your right leg where there's a cramp, and you slide down it (maybe even going "wheeeee") and drop off exactly where the cells or muscles are that you need to talk to.

So now let's do that. Pick a place in your body that has been giving you trouble and decide which pathway out of your room will take you there. Hook yourself on to the nerve and slide into the tunnel. Ride the nerve (or artery or vein, if you wish) down to the location and step off to greet your crew.

Step 3. Listen, Apologize, Be Honest

When you arrive at your destination, remember to be completely honest. You are the captain, and maybe these particular crewmembers are looking for succor in their time of fear and trouble, or maybe they just need a good pep talk. You will be able to tell. (Whatever you determine after you've been there a few minutes will be correct. Remember, there is no wrong way to do this.) Just as you carefully observed – visualized – the numbers earlier, and saw the detail in your launch room, now look at the cells and organs, muscles or bones, etc., that you have come to see.

However you see them is okay, just make sure you see and sense them, whatever they look like.

Now begin a dialogue with them, as if they are your good and faithful friends; you began this voyage together and you've come to check up on them and get reacquainted. And, if they are angry or afraid, you're there to make things right. Again, talk out loud, and imagine what they are saying back to you. It can – and probably will – be an inane conversation. Have the dialogue, listen to it, *but do not edit what is being said*. Let your imagination fly, carry on as if you and they were old drinking buddies. What I usually hear is, "It's about time you got down here."

Step 4: Repair, Physically and Psychologically

Whatever you experience there, act on it, now. If they need help, give them help. If they need fixing, you've got all the tools in your back pocket that you need to fix them right then and there. If they need a hug, give them several. And if they need to let off steam, listen. If they need you to apologize for neglecting them, do it, from the bottom of your heart. And mean it when you say you won't neglect them again. After all, they are your friends, your partners, your crew on this amazing experience, and they contribute to making it possible.

Sometimes I imagine I'm a telephone repairman, splicing into a damaged wire and repairing the connections – the wire being my gestalt of a nerve or an artery, for example. Sometimes I'll decide that some imaginary "control box" is responsible for a muscle or group of muscles, and if I have observed that they're uptight or not operating very smoothly, I'll open it up and fix something to let a bit more energy flow, or I'll exercise a switch or dial, to remove some corrosion that's collected over the years.

You can imagine anything in your mind. And when you fix something there, so what? You haven't affected anyone but yourself, have you? Of course, that is a question for another book.

Step 5: Insist, Love, Cajole, Coach

Imagine what you would say if you were the coach of a football team that was getting creamed out there on the field, and you had ignored the game and walked into the locker room to make a phone call. Now you're back, and they have needed you. Be there for them. Be the coach – the captain of the ship. Whatever love and encouragement they need, give it to them, they trust you.

Step 6: Give Thanks

Spend as much time with your crew as you need, until you completely understand that all is well between you, and they are comfortable going back to their perfect function.

Then thank them for the wonderful job they do for you, and say goodbye, promising to always be there for them, and frequently in touch. Let them know they can count on you from now on, now that you know that you can communicate with them like this.

As you leave them to return to their perfect functioning, know that it's done, and give thanks also to that which created you for the knowledge you have, and for the new reality of a perfectly functioning body. Then you may move to another part of your body, or slowly return to the launch room, greeting other parts of your crew as you move by them, stopping if and when you wish, to chat and thank them for their excellent work – out loud.

Step 7: Release and Know

Once you have returned to your launch room, look around it again, seeing once again just where everything is (you can decorate it with anything you wish on your next trip), then turn out the lights if you wish, and step into your elevator.

Ride the elevator back up to the top, and step out into your starry space again. Now, as you look around, you may realize that this space is actually the inside of the medulla oblongata of your brain – the part that connects the brain to the spinal cord. All you need do now is expand your awareness to fill out your brain completely, and you're back home. You can stay there for awhile if you want to, noticing how it feels. Then you may open your eyes whenever you wish.

Now forget everything that just happened, and go do something else. It might help to say aloud, "It's done, and I release it to be."

Step 8: Now Go Do Something Else Fun

It's important to remember to go play. This entire process works best when it's approached as play, especially the dialogue with your body. Friends play together. If you see something that could mean illness, treat it like it's no more than a bothersome "irregularity" in the cells and wash it away with a rag, or pull out some oil from your back pocket and lubricate it, or whatever you playfully feel it needs, playfully give it. And it's done.

Most of all, don't expect any immediate change. You might, on occasion, feel differently afterward, but usually noticeable changes take some time, especially in the beginning. It's almost as if the universe is testing us, to see if we really accept this, or we're demanding immediate results or we want our money back. Don't look for immediate results. KNOW that it is done, *in the face of no evidence*. The results will come when you're not paying attention.

Well, then, there you are. Those are the rudiments of the full process. Obviously, as you play with it over time, it will become easier, and faster. Soon you won't have to do the entire counting thing, you'll just jump down to whatever hurts, see yourself standing beside it, tools in hand, and start to talk. But you see from my own experiences that too often we forget to use it, even when we know perfectly well how.

THE SHORT WAY
Quickie phrases that work for me

For bumps, scrapes, cuts and other painful would-be injuries:

"*Not a word of truth to it,*" followed by a quick trip inside the injury to tell the cells: "Hey you guys, bet that scared you, didn't it? Well, you're fine, everything's just fine…" etc.

For potentially larger problems:

"*I am perfect health. I know that my (leg, arm, etc.) is fine. I thought I was injured but I was just mistaken…*" followed by the process.

My experience is that when I do this I actually have to give up being injured. I can't have it both ways. I always conclude that it *looked* like this was going to be a big injury, but actually I was wrong, it was very small, or even nothing at all. "Sure got lucky that time!" I often say.

Who was it said "Never trade luck for skill"?

◊

Chapter XII: Take Your Healing Where You Find It

There is a joke you've probably heard about the pious man who got caught in a flood. In the middle of the night, the police came knocking on the man's door, telling him to evacuate, the area would soon be flooded. But he refused, saying, "God will save me."

By morning, the water had risen several feet higher, surging into the first floor of his house. A fireman floating down the street in a boat offered him a ride to safety, but the man still refused, saying, "God will save me."

By noon the flood had forced the man to the roof of his house, when a helicopter arrived and lowered a rope ladder for him to climb up. "No," said the man, "God will save me."

Not long after, the flood sweeps the entire house away, and the man drowns. Upon discovering he's standing before the Pearly Gates, the man stomps around, furious. God notices this and approaches the man. "What's wrong, my son?" he asked.

"What's wrong!? Everything! You said you'd save me and you let me drown, that's what's wrong!"

God replies, "I didn't let you drown. I sent you a rescue team to evacuate you, and you refused it. I sent you a boat, and you refused it. Finally I sent you a helicopter, and you refused it. Only then did you drown."

We may have our hearts so completely set on magical/miraculous cures for our special disease or problem that we completely ignore the perfectly fine but mundane solution staring us right in the face. Don't make that mistake. Every cure for disease is a miracle, and every cure for disease is mundane. The only difference is time, place and attitude. In 1940 penicillin was a miracle. Today it's not just mundane. If a doctor gave you penicillin for something you'd probably think he was too old to practice medicine.

A hundred years ago aspirin was a miracle drug. By the end of the 20th century, we'd become so bored with it that we'd concocted knock-offs so we didn't have to take "mere aspirin" anymore - but it was still a miracle drug. A hundred and fifty years ago nitrous oxide ("laughing gas"), still commonly used in dental surgery today, was not only a miracle, it was so amazing that the Harvard Medical School refused to believe it even worked. But even today it eliminates pain so well that operations can be performed that were impossible before.

Don't wait for a miracle. Accept as your particular miracle whatever shows up and fixes your ailment, even if it doesn't come wrapped in the pretty little miracle package you hoped it would come in.

Put simply, if you talk to your body and practice the focused process of this book, and then find a mundane medical practitioner (that's "doctor," for short) down the street who can help cure your ailment, be happy, you've succeeded. If the cure only comes from some occult healer you've found deep in the Amazon who paints you with monkey dung, great, live long and prosper. It is not ours to know How, only to know That.

Accept the healing that comes, no matter from where. What was it we learned in Sunday school, catechism and the Torah (to name a few)? All things are equal in God's sight. This includes successful methods of healing.

Besides, here's my two cents: Our experience of "be-ing" doesn't stop at the edge of our skin. Everything that happens to us "in here" and "out there" is all part of us, part of our particular and personal universe, and there is no difference between the two except in the way we apply our limited ability to perceive. We define the difference, just as academics down through the centuries have defined chemistry as different from physics, and music as different from electronics. They all use the same basic information and building blocks, just perceived and applied in different ways.

A Theory

When we talk to our body, we are creating a crack in the universe wherein we inject the concept that our apparently sick body might in fact actually be whole and healed. Proved long ago with the early remote viewing experiments, and theorized long before that by quantum physics – and Buddhism and Hinduism ages earlier – this powerful concept we have thought up, and spoken aloud, doesn't stop reverberating at the inside edge of our skin, but rather it travels into all of "reality," across the gaps between the electrons and protons of "our" atoms and into and across those atoms we do not normally accept as "ours," such as those in the air, for example.

And that concept, that Word, as it were, continues, faster than the speed of light, all at once permeating the world and the universe, and its very existence changes things. That which might have been without the Word being spoken is changed to favor that which we have imagined *might* be, insisted might be, commanded to be, and thus a very slight bit of extra emphasis is given the potential outcome, the potential future, which we have imagined for ourselves and declared into this Word.

And if it is necessary for the perfect fulfillment of the Universal Plan that a doctor or a scientist or an Amazon medicine man or the lady next door should announce their discovery of the cure for your illness, then they will, and you will hear of it, and be healed. And if it is within the grand plan that a slight shift takes place in your body in order for your healing to occur, and nothing more, then it is possible that that is what will happen.

I repeat:

**IT IS NOT OUR BUSINESS TO KNOW <u>HOW</u>,
IT IS ONLY FOR US TO KNOW <u>THAT</u>.**

There's No Such Thing as a Wrong Healing

A few years ago I started feeling pain in my abdomen and discovered a growth in my scrotum that scared the hell out of me. Remember, I'm the son and grandson of hypochondriacs, so I'm sure that any small anomaly in my body is quickly going to grow to become cancer, heart disease, stroke, or a combination of all three.

This wasn't a small anomaly, it was a pretty good-sized one, and I was terrified. I quickly read up on testicular cancer, the disease that can kill, and although I was in my 50's and this disease affects men under 30, I *knew* I had it. And I knew it was spreading minute by minute throughout my body as I sat there! I could "feel its tentacles." It's a good thing our thoughts and imaginings are not all manifest, or hypochondriacs like me would have been dead of ten different diseases years ago.

Why is it we can imagine perfectly that terrible diseases are overtaking us, but it's so hard to imagine perfect health happening? Because perfect health is our normal state of being, and it's only when we think we aren't in perfect health that we take notice. What's to imagine about boring old good health? That's like going to a movie where nothing happens. Yawn.

Well, with this growth occupying my every waking thought, I wanted to see a doctor, but before facing what I might be told by the meat doctors ("Hey, there's a growth there, let's cut it out and hit you with some chemo and radiation!"), I felt I needed some real inner strength, so I checked myself into the Optimum Health Institute in San Diego for a "cleaning out" – physical and spiritual.

They really do the job, starting on day one when you no longer drink coffee (my addiction), soft drinks or tea, or eat anything containing fat, sugar, salt or a long list of other things that comprise 99% of our daily diet. I left a half-eaten bag of potato chips and some cookies in the car, thinking I'd sneak out and finish one day while I was there...what a joke.

The diet for the duration consists of such delectables as puréed watermelon rind (that's breakfast), juiced cucumbers, kelp, mung bean and other fun sprouts and, on day four after a three-day juice fast, real applesauce (whoopee!).

It's essentially a vegan diet, with heavy emphasis on live, sprouted foods, fresh from the ground. No animal foods, no milk, no eggs, no wheat. Nothing is heated over 105 degrees F, and over the years they've developed a surprising variety of recipes that actually taste pretty good – once you lose your hunger for caffeine, sugar and animal fat – saturated, hydrogenated or what-have-you.

Oh, and then there's their central staple, wheat grass juice. It's locally grown, of course, cut and juiced by each guest, and taken at ten, two and four – at least. And inserted into practically every orifice of your body twice a day. There are wheat grass poultices for tumors and wounds; stick some up your nose for allergies, in your ears for ear aches, between your toes for athletes foot. And of course, the *pièce de résistance,* the wheat grass enema for everything else that ails you.

A shock to the psyche, to be sure, but it works. After a couple weeks, it's amazing how wonderful you feel (and how much weight you lose!) They work on your psyche, too, and on your heart – the spiritual one – treating you as a whole person, not just a physical body with something to fix. There are classes on spirituality and love and breathing and meditation and coming to terms with life. They know that terminal cancer patients often show up there after doctors have given up hope, and they leave no stone unturned in helping them.

Terminal patients go there to save their lives; aware people go there to cleanse preventatively. I went there to talk to my body. I didn't want to have cancer, I wanted to have something normal and extremely benign. I much prefer being a hypochondriac to actually being ill.

During the day there was plenty of time to sit quietly and rest, read, or just meditate. I took advantage of it, found a private space, and directed my attention to the pain in my belly and below. We talked. It told me that I had coughed too much when I had a chest infection in the spring, and I realized I probably had a hernia. I asked it to fix itself. Why couldn't the tear in the tissue reconnect back to normal? In those two weeks, it didn't.

I went lower, and with great trepidation connected with that large third thing in my scrotum. I asked it what it was and would it please not harm me. It didn't reply. My little scuba-suited me (Mini-Me?) crawled around and through it, telling it how much I appreciated it coming, and promising I'd learn whatever lesson it had for me. But would it please now go away, diminish; return to be a part of the universe. Unlike that mole years ago, no response. I worked on it for two weeks and found that from time to time I could get it smaller, to maybe even 20% of its original size, but it always returned to normal when I left it alone for awhile. What was I doing wrong, I wondered.

When I returned home, I stayed on the diet and made an appointment with the best urologist I could find. Between then and the date of the office visit I spent much time talking to my body, reminding it that I loved it, even that part which terrified me, and I began to relent somewhat, renegotiating with it, telling the growth that it was okay to stick around so long as it didn't harm me.

By the time I got my appointment with the urologist, I had decided this "thing" was actually an implant done by visitors from outer space so they could eavesdrop on my sex life. (I'd been watching too much Star Trek again, I think.) It took me six weeks to get to the urologist since I first discovered the "thing," and it took the urologist all of two minutes to confirm that my alien implant was a common "spermatocele," an innocuous collection of sperm from over the years that had not made its way out the normal pathway.

"Leave it alone," he advised, "it's meaningless, they're pretty common."

So! Lots of guys have alien implants in their scrota, eh!? Now we know their secret! I wonder what they're finding out about us. For a few days after the visit to the doctor I felt so giddy that I started talking into my scrotum late at night. "Hello there, can you hear me? Are you guys getting the information you wanted?"

But what had I wanted, a miracle cure or perfect health? I left the doctor's office in perfect health – just as I had gone in, by the way. But the little "thing" was still there. Had I been healed or not? Did I ever have anything to be healed about?

Or had all that conversing with my body changed the course of my physical condition? Was there a time prior when this diagnosis might have been different, and my thoughts, actions and words had effected a change in the direction?

It's possible. We'll never know. What I did certainly didn't hurt anything.

But there's more: The urologist also diagnosed my hernia, and told me that at some time or other in the future I might want to have it fixed. Six months later, after living with the debilitation for awhile, and still not being successful at "self-repair," I looked into surgery, and found a simple laparoscopy technique that could have me in and out in a few hours. If I couldn't fix it myself, that seemed like a pretty cool alternative.

When I went for the pre-op visit to the surgeon, he asked me if I had considered a vasectomy, since it would be an easy snip while he was "in there." My wife and I had been discussing this very thing, and so I said yes. Then he noticed the spermatocele and said casually, "Oh, and this will go away after the vasectomy."

Duh!

Remember the third part of the process, "Release"? I had long since released my healing intention on that thing in my scrotum, after putting an amazing amount of energy into having it go away. And now it was all but gone, except for the manifestation part. And now that would come.

This stuff works, in spite of time and space and our doubts. And even after all these years, I'm still amazed every time.

Remember, we are not an island standing apart from the rest of reality. That which we put into deliberate intention changes things, sets them in motion, within and without, because in truth there is no difference between that which is "us" and that which is "not us."

If I talk to my body and ask it to heal itself, and next week a new medical technique turns up that fixes my problem (and I go have the procedure done), I HAVE RECEIVED MY HEALING! I never learned this lesson more convincingly than by a later experience with an ophthalmologist – see Epilogue.

We are not alone in the universe. We are one with it.

◊

Chapter XIII: Out of the Closet

As I have been writing this book, I have become acutely aware of the fact that its publication will clearly bring me "out of the closet" with my philosophy and belief structure. Until now, I have hidden behind my basic anonymity as just another innocuous 'name in the phone book,' and only talked in general terms with close friends about the process of sitting in a quiet room (or noisy freeway) and talking aloud to my body. While feeling that this is something that could help everyone, I've been loathe to admit to many people that I practice it myself.

I knew that if I published this book, I had to come to terms with the fact that my secret was out, and I'd be asked about it all the time, by friends, strangers, and particularly by antagonists. To paraphrase an old adage, "no good idea goes unpunished," and I'd better be ready.

My time of hiding ended even before the book was finished. We were on a family trip over a holiday weekend, visiting friends in the country, and the kids were invited to swim in a nearby pond. They readily accepted, and we tagged along to keep an eye on them.

There were probably 75 people there, mostly strangers to each other, but friends of our hosts. The 20 or so children played around a large wooden pontoon raft probably 20 feet square, secured by ropes at the water's edge. Moved by the waves created by all the kids in the water, the raft floated into the muddy bank and out again, until its ropes jerked taut, which would yank it slowly back against the bank once again to repeat the process. Getting on and off it required timing the raft's movement so as not to miss it.

That's where my problem arose. After lunch I walked down to the water's edge to jump on the raft and chat with a friend who was relaxing on it. The top of the raft was about three feet above the bank, and as I started to hop up onto it, it floated away from me just enough that I landed heel-first on the top and that foot slid forward on the wet surface, right out from under me.

My back leg didn't make it all the way onto the raft, it slammed hard against the top edge and then, bearing all my weight, slid down the side of the raft and stuck into the mud below. At that moment the heavy raft reached the end of its tether and started back toward the bank – me with one leg on the raft and the other stuck in the mud below. Before I could extricate my stuck leg the raft slammed into it just below the knee. I heard a loud crack – everyone nearby heard it – someone screamed and I immediately went into automatic.

All I remember after that was that I waited until the raft sloshed forward again and then I pulled my leg out of the mud. Somehow I hopped up onto the raft and pulled my leg into my chest, wrapped my hands around the open wound and closed my eyes. I remember knowing that I was (a) not going to look at the wound, and (b) no one else was going to either. I also remember realizing that if I expected to walk away from that place and drive home, I was going to have to "do my thing" right there in front of God and everybody. No more hiding in the closet.

So I did. With my eyes closed, I put my mind's attention down my leg all the way to the cells in the skin and bone, and I started talking. I remember hearing myself say something like, "You guys are fine...I'm sorry you got such a scare, but everything's okay, and you're fine." I was deep in my leg, right where those terrified cells were hiding. They were going to hear from the Captain, now, and they were going to be fine. They WERE ALREADY fine.

I also remember feeling my shin bone right at the spot it hit the corner of the raft, and recognizing a deep indentation in the bone that wasn't there before. And I remember being afraid. And then refusing that fear, and talking all the louder to my leg.

INSIDE my leg. "I know this scared you, but you're perfectly fine, you're wonderful, and I love you."

By that time several people had gathered around, probably concerned as much for my mental state as my physical one, and one asked me if I was okay – to which I replied, "Absolutely fine, I'm just reminding my leg that everything's okay. It'll take me a few minutes, but everything's fine." He asked to see the wound. I refused, telling him that whatever he might see was from the past, not from what was now, and the "now' condition of my leg was just in my mind, and he would have to trust me that it was okay. I don't know if he understood, but I didn't care, I was busy washing away centuries of instinct at that moment and I didn't want anyone reminding me of what was "supposed" to be.

Yes, I felt the bone, and I still knew it was *not* broken, not even bent, in spite of probability, because its cells now fully realized that they were in good hands.

Ten, maybe fifteen minutes passed, before I came out of my completely focused state and took my hands away from my leg. As I did, I reminded myself that what I would see was what "had been," an eternity of nanoseconds ago, but what was NOW was a perfect leg, with perhaps a bit of scraped skin as a reminder of the experience. After all, if people didn't see anything, they might think I really was nuts, sitting there doing all that talking to my leg while apparently nothing had really happened to me. Interesting.

Someone asked me if I wanted to go to the hospital, and I said no. He gave me a hand getting off the raft, and then I finally looked at my leg. There was a long section of skin that had been abraded, like a skinned knee, where my leg had slid down the edge of the raft, and it was bleeding a little here and there. That was all. I put pressure on it, felt around with my hands, and the bone was completely intact. Not even tender. And what surprised me the most, there was only a slight indentation where 15 minutes ago there had been a hell of a lot lot more. (Maybe that's the definition of "hell" after all – the worst that could be, but doesn't have to be.)

Someone else offered me an antibiotic swab, warning me of the dangers of infection from the pond water, and I used it, then found a bandage in the car and taped it over the skinned area, "So no one becomes squeamish," I lied.

I enjoyed the rest of the day at the pond, walking on the leg *knowing* it was normal, and when we pulled up stakes and returned home that night, I took a shower, cleaned the wound, rebandaged it, and went to bed. Next day, the bone was sore, but there was no bruising, and the contusion was healing perfectly. I walked two miles that day, and ran three the next, frequently reminding my leg that it was fine, and telling the cells just how proud I was of them for handling that scary experience so well.

Three days later the bandage came off, and all was back to normal. It took more than a month for a reddish area the size of a quarter to disappear. I decided that was to continually remind me of what happened. I keep my wildly bent spoons on my desk for the same reason.

Ironically, after all my timidness at doing it in public, half a dozen people at the pond came up to me and mentioned how moved they were at how I handled it. "I thought sure your leg was broken!" they'd say, "I can't believe all you have is a little abrasion!"

I didn't tell them that somewhere inside I was wondering what would happen when I talked to my leg. But I played the game in the face of no evidence, and I won. WE won.

Even today, years later, there's a small indentation in the shin bone just below the knee. I'm glad to have it. It reminds me that this process works.

Don't Forget to Use It!

No matter how much you supposedly know about what to do with an injury, you still forget. I always think that's my old self still wanting life to be the way I used to think it was – I was not responsible for anything, life just "happened." So don't expect to remember to use it very often in the beginning – or in my case, even 20 years after you've begun. The other night I was I was hacksawing a piece of metal in the garage for a little project I was working on.

Of course, when you cut metal, it leaves sharp edges, and I was nonchalantly sliding my fingers along the metal to see if there were actually sharp edges there when a sharp pain in my finger signaled "yes, there are, stupid." Too late, I realized that maybe I should have checked with my eyes instead. There were lots of sharp edges on the metal, and one of them sliced a nice half-inch nick in my fingertip.

I grabbed the cut and washed it, not even thinking to talk to it. Then the phone rang, and by the time I hung up the cut was forgotten, I was tired, so I went to bed. I had just turned out the light when my cut yelled up at me that it was there, still unattended to.

My wife was asleep beside me, I couldn't remember where we keep the bandages, but I knew we had some super glue in the bathroom, so I rolled out of bed, grabbed the glue, held the cut closed with my thumb, and dabbed a drop on the cut. In seconds it would be bonded closed, and that would get me through the night. I turned out the light and headed back to bed.

Then, halfway across the room, I realized I'd better make sure I hadn't stuck my thumb and finger together with the crazy stuff – I'd done that before, too. I pulled them apart – well I tried to, and discovered to my frustration that I'd done it again. Some of the glue had run down my finger and collected in the crack where my thumb was pressed up against it. If you believe the superglue label, my thumb and forefinger were now bonded forever.

It was very late, so my first thought was, I'd just let them stick that way for a couple days until nature took its course, and my skin shed enough cells to unstick them. Then I decided that wasn't a good idea, I'd better get them apart now, which meant going downstairs, getting a new single-edged razor blade out of the kitchen, heating it over the stove to sterilize it, getting a magnifying glass, setting myself under a bright light and slicing away, trying to avoid any nerve-bearing dermis. (Is there a solvent for this stuff? I've never seen it.)

When I got settled with a razor and looked seriously at the job ahead, I thought again of waiting until morning and going to the doctor. The glued area was nearly an inch long, and probably 3/8" wide. Big. At the doctor's I'd get a shot of xylocaine or something to kill the inevitable pain of slicing into my fingers with a sharp blade.

Then I realized I didn't want to be that embarrassed, so I started the dreaded slicing.

Needless to say, with almost every slice I hit a nerve. I'm the sort of guy whose threshold of pain is crossed when a nurse enters the room holding the needle she's going to be putting in my arm…so you can understand how completely out of the realm of reality it is for me to contemplate slicing my own finger with a razor blade. I've never been a good candidate for any kind of drug you have to put in your own arm with a syringe; I don't think I'd make a very good diabetic, even. 'Short-lived' would probably describe me.

Anyway, after 15 minutes of slicing and dicing, wincing and yelping, while my poor wife lay in bed (now awake) wishing she could do something to help me or shut me up, I had gotten about one-tenth of the way through the glued area. This was not working out. Then, finally remembering what I should have thought of much earlier, I said to myself, "it's amazing how easily and painlessly this razor cuts through the rest of this glue. Now my fingers are going to come apart quickly and easily." And, for good measure, "With every cut, this blade is going to part the dried glue, not even touching my skin, and I'm going to be done in no time."

And the amazing thing was, that it was so. While it had taken me 15 painful minutes to get the first ten percent cut through, the remaining 90% came apart in less than two minutes. With no more pain. Even as I was saying the words, I watched in amazement as they began coming true.

Then I laughed, because it's fun to still be that little kid who is amazed that this stuff works.

◊

*O Death! thou dunnest of all duns!
Thou daily knockest at doors…*

- Lord Byron, "Don Juan"

Chapter XIV: Talk to Your Body About Your Death

Well, who's going to share the experience besides you two? You one, that is. In our culture, we tend to put all our emphasis on living, and in particular, on being (and staying) young, shunning the subject of death as if it were, well, Death.

But many other cultures have dealt with the matter of dying quite directly. For example, the "Tibetan Book of the Dead" was used for centuries to assist the dying to cross into the next state of being while still completely conscious. Much time and intense training was spent by Buddhist practitioners in preparation for the experience of death.

According to the ancient text, death begins with a gradual process of dissolution of the senses and energies that worked in cooperation with physical consciousness. These dissolutions are experienced partially in our normal sleep, and are said to be consciously generated in meditation by students of advanced yoga; but only at the time of death are they experienced both completely and, of course, inevitably. When Buddhist practitioners become skilled in inducing the dissolution phases at will, they gain the ability to apply the same techniques during sleep, and ultimately during the first moments of dying.

Talk about control of your life. Where's the terror if you are involved that completely in the process? There isn't any.

In my approach to dealing with our bodies, I can't figure out for the life of me why some kind of discussion isn't held about it between the most important parties to this most important event of your life, you and your body. I mean, you would have at least one pre-departure chat with a companion taking a trip a hundred miles across the state, and maybe even a lengthy preparatory immersion in the culture and language of an exotic land you're about to visit, so why can't you have a serious conversation about taking this monumental trip, with the vehicle that's most particularly involved in the experience, your body?

Maybe you can't sit in the lotus position for ten years and chant *Om*. Okay, well, how about something like drifting down into that space you created in your mind, looking straight into your body's eyes man-to-body (woman-to-body?) and saying, "Hey, you know, I'm scared shitless to die, and you're the one who's going to cause it to happen."??

In truth, don't be surprised to hear back, "I'M the one? Who fed me all that chocolate chip cookie dough ice cream late at night for so many years? I'd be working fine into your second century if you weren't so impossibly stupid about taking care of me!"

However you start the dialogue, begin. You're just talking, after all.

Don't we all want an easy, painless death? Why not discuss this with your body? Who better? Why not have a conversation about how scared you are that it's just going to up and quit on you some Monday morning[20] without warning, or contract some painfully slow but always fatal disease, and you'll wind up in the cancer ward begging for stronger and stronger drugs…WHY NOT?

This kind of conversation is certainly not going to hurt you. And if nothing else happens, it will ease your mind a bit, as you get out in the open that terrible little secret most of us carry around – that we're scared out of our wits to die.

And then again, you might be surprised. Who knows, you might just find a place of at-one-ment with your closest friend, and work out a way to exit this mortal coil easily…fearlessly, even.

It's possible.

◊

---

[20] The American Medical Association says that's when most heart attacks happen.

Chapter XV: Now It's Your Turn

Why don't we talk to ourselves like this? Why don't we address our best, most intimate partner – our body – the way we commonly talk to our best friend, our lover, our child? It's right under our nose, after all!

We meditate ourselves to greater peace and health, guide ourselves to the Light, pray hard for health and a better life, read all the books on stress reduction, better eating, lowering cholesterol. We'll try the all-cookie diet, the all Diet Pepsi diet, we'll march to free the radicals and oxymorons (I get confused after awhile), let strangers with medical degrees poke and test our bodies, tell our deepest secrets to psychologists and psychiatrists, but we never ever address that monster in the closet, that marvel of sophisticated bioengineering that brought and keeps us here...even when it screams for attention!

What do you think a backache is, anyway, or a pain in the knee, or heart disease, for that matter? If you were Captain Kirk, and the engine started acting up, you'd be down there in a second talking to Scotty, wouldn't you? Of course you would. You'd be derelict in your duty otherwise.

But let our heart start to give us a pain, and we freak, freeze, and either ignore it or head for a doctor. WHY DON'T WE SIT DOWN AND TALK TO IT? Why don't we get down there and find out what the complaint is? "Hey, knee, I see you've got a problem. What's going on?"

Know the answer you'll get? Something like, *"Damn, it's about time you got down out of your ivory tower and came to see us! We've been down here bustin' our butt for years and you've never come to find out how we're doing! Give us a break! We do all the heavy lifting and you sit up there ignoring us!"*

How do you diffuse an angry, frustrated part of your crew who feels ignored and unappreciated? Well, maybe you just sit down and apologize. Maybe you say, "You know what, you're right. I was not aware that that I could even do this."

Maybe you 'mother' them a bit: "But I'm here now, and I want you to know that I love you, and I appreciate you. You are so incredibly important to me, and to everyone on this ship, that I'm really sorry I haven't told you until now." Then go around to everyone there and hug them, and tell them truthfully just how much you appreciate their incredible work—because you certainly know you do! – and promise to never ignore them again.

Then, ask what you can do for them. And listen, they'll tell you. Don't expect the answer to necessarily be in words – you're the wordmeister, the brain, the captain. But you will KNOW what they are telling you, because you have connected with them – with this part of your spaceship – and communication will happen.

Love is the key. Every part of your body needs to know you love it. Just as members of a team look to the captain for encouragement, guidance and support, every part of your body, the muscles, organs, and cells, look to "you," the captain, for their nourishment. You know that thing that coaches do with their players before every game? – The "everyone holds hands and says 'Yea Team!'" thing? Why don't you do that once in awhile? Zip a blast of God-light down into your body and say, "Yea Team!" Gives me a chill just thinking about it!

Ever heard of dogs who won't eat until their master comes home? I'm convinced parts of our bodies don't want to function well until they know they're loved, they're safe, and they're appreciated.

SO TELL THEM!

And why can't we do this everyday? Maybe we can. Let's find out. All we have to do is listen to – feel – our bodies. They're always saying something. The whole team inside making this incredible journey with us needs regular attention, acknowledgement, care, concern, love. A crew that is openly and honest appreciated will never mutiny – and they will always work hard and well for you.

When something feels wrong, don't be afraid. Somebody down there is just trying to get your attention, sending you a message: "Hey up there on the bridge, pay attention, I need you!" Sit down, close your eyes, and "go" there. Start by apologizing that you haven't been around for awhile – they're usually feeling neglected. Talk to your cells as if they were your hardworking friends, with whom you've embarked on this wonderful journey. Pat them on the back for a job well done, and remind them just how important they are to you – out of love and appreciation, not fear. A hug wouldn't hurt, either. They'll relax, and work miracles for you.

Make regular visits around the ship. The good captain always visits the crew, just to check in and see how everyone's doing. When you do that, if there's a need, it will come up. You'll get it communicated to you. And however strange you may think it seems to others, or however afraid you are of being seen doing this, ignore those fears and go with it. I just remember that if I had a cell phone to my ear and were whisked back to 1850 while talking on it, I'd quickly be put in an insane asylum. Every new idea is always crazy in the beginning.

Speaking of crazy, like most people, I had two grandmothers; they both were alive when I was a kid. One was a hypochondriac, as you know, and the other one talked to St. Peter and St. John, who she always saw standing beside me whenever I went to visit her…in the State Mental Institution in Alexandria, Louisiana. Was she crazy, or were we, for putting her there just because we couldn't see them? Galileo went to jail for believing the earth was round, too. Maybe my grandmother was mentally ill, maybe she was just ahead of her time. The preconceptions of the observer affect the reality of the observation, remember?

Now if you'll excuse me, there's a little floater in my eye that's starting to like being the center of my attention. The eye doctor says "get used to it, it comes with age." Huh. I need to go have a chat with it. (Sing with me now, Blondie's big '80s hit: *"One way, or another, I'm gonna getcha, I'm gonna getcha getcha getcha…"*)

THE END
(for now)

Epilogue: Working With The Doctor
The Floater Story

For the years since my threatened loss of sight in my right eye, my vision has been remarkably good, amazingly good, actually, "for my age." I have retained right at 20/30 vision in both eyes and an ability to read without glasses in all but the dimmest light, even though I turned 60 while writing this book.

Not that I always had perfect vision. At age 12 I was diagnosed with classic myopia – nearsightedness, and wore glasses for 17 years, which, ironically, kept me from attending the Air Force Academy to become a fighter pilot (my childhood dream), just before the outbreak of the Vietnam War. My local Congressman had nominated me to the Academy, and I went for the physical exam, where I learned that because of my then 20/40 vision the Air Force would not permit me to be a jet jockey. Immediately I demurred on the appointment and enrolled in a civilian university.

When I finally did do military service in Vietnam, it was in an air conditioned radio station in Saigon, far away from the front lines. While I was there, fighter pilots like I had wanted to be were frequently being shot down in enemy territory. If they survived, they wound up in the Hanoi Hilton or dead. Think John McCain, among many others. Looking back, I often wondered who had been looking out for me.

When I was 24, living in Miami after the Army and college, I broke my glasses one day, and had to find a new optometrist and get a new prescription. After a standard eye exam confirming my nearsightedness, he suggested that he could possibly cure it! He told me he had a theory that many people like me had what he called *pseudomyopia*, from too much close reading when we were young. Now, no one I knew had ever heard of pseudomyopia in those years, but he promised his treatment wouldn't make my eyes worse, so I said, "Why not?"[21] He figured it would take four to five years, and if successful, I might not need glasses again until presbyopia (farsightedness) would set in years later.

Over the next five years I went to him for an annual checkup, and each year my eyes improved slightly. Each time, he would change my prescription, giving me glasses that were always just slightly weaker than would be normally called for, forcing my eyes to work and get stronger. He also gave me eye and neck exercises to do twice a day, every day. Each time I got new glasses, my eyes would work so hard that I had headaches for three to four weeks afterward. But sure enough, by my 29th birthday, my vision was 20/20 in both eyes. And thus they remained for many years before very slowly relaxing into the slight myopia I have now.

But a few months ago I woke up to a strange image. I had been working hard, and putting myself under a great deal of stress to prove something special with a project I was doing. I came home on a Friday night exhausted, stressed, irritable, and feverish and went to bed. Saturday morning I woke up with a sharp pain in my right eye – yes, *that* right eye. The spider-web right eye that Jack Houck reminded me was perfect years ago.

When I got up, I realized that I could see an irregular circle inside the eye that floated across my field of vision when I moved my eye. At first I went for a long run, and tried the "not a word of truth to it" speech. Then I sat in a hot tub and talked to the "thing," just as I had talked to the mole and spermatocele and leg and heart over the years. But nothing intelligible came from it. I tried for two days to deal with it using every trick I've taught you in this book, but nothing worked. It stayed there, bugging the heck out of my heretofore perfect vision.

Monday morning I made an appointment with an ophthalmologist, and hit the internet search engines.

---

[21] Over the years that's become my mantra…"Why not?" It leads to interesting experiences.

It was actually called a *floater*, I learned, due to a post vitreous detachment – "something that comes with age to 70% of us," the first ophthalmologist who looked at it told me. The learned doctor also said, "Get used to it, there's nothing we can do."

Oh, oh. There they were again, those magic words! *There's Nothing We Can Do.* Well, reinvigorated, I thought "Ha, there may be nothing YOU can do, but I know something to do!" and went home and started my talking process all over again. Just like my father taught me, "The difficult we do right away, the impossible takes a little longer." After the experiences with my mole, and my heart, and my daughter, and half a hundred other times when I've used this technique, I figured in spite of the problem over the weekend I'd have this pest out of my eye in no time.

So I went into my mental room and mediated and slid up beside it and talked to the thing. I cajoled and commanded. I summoned up angels and anyone else "out there" who might be interested in helping (you never know who's listening!). I talked to my metaphysical friends. And through it all that irregular ring stayed right where it was – zinging in and out of my field of focus every time I moved my eye.

Damn.

I looked for possibilities, and found one. A brilliant ocular surgeon in Santa Monica took one look in my eye and said, "Oh, that's a Weiss ring," the part of the vitreous that used to be attached around the optic nerve. Apparently the vitreous gel in our eyes over time becomes a bit less gelatinous, and can pull away from the inner surface of the eye, allowing the eye to see the little "clumps of collagen" where contact with the retina had once been. He could get it out in 20 minutes, he said, by a vitrectomy, surgically removing the vitreous gel and replacing it with a viscous saline solution.

That of course would require three "penetrations" of the eyeball, by two operating instruments and a lighted microscope. Oh, and when I was done, I'd have maybe a year of crystal clear vision, and then the lens would begin to cloud over (as a reaction to the brute force attack, I suppose, they don't know why yet), and it was certain a cataract would form on the lens. That, of course, would require operation number two. Amazing medicine certainly – cataract surgery these days is fairly routine – but I didn't want to make it elective surgery. Not yet, anyway.

Then I found another possibility, besides the "do it yourself" method described in this book and which I was still diligently pursuing (maybe it was that very diligence that was causing me trouble?). There is in medical use a device known as a YAG Laser, so named because of the chemicals it uses to fire it.[22] I researched its use for quite a while, and read that (a) it often makes many little bothersome particles out of the big bothersome particles it breaks up, and (b) there is still some concern about lens clouding with it, apparently because it is an intense focused light aimed right at the lens, after all. So nix on that one, too.

But my biggest problem was not that medicine might be able to do something for me, it was that I thought I might need it to. Even after the experience with the hernia, there was something particularly troublesome about needing help with my eyes. "Seeing clearly." "Vision." Something about the multiple meanings of these words reverberated through my being. What was going on here? Remember what I said in the beginning of this book, "Use all the tools in the toolbox when the time comes."? I wasn't doing that. I was still supposing that I could heal myself all by myself, when in truth I had the world at my disposal.

I thought about all this for a long time. Months, in fact, while I lived with Dr. Weiss's grand floater in my eye. Then I started the search again for a solution. My conversations with my

---

[22] The YAG laser is a solid state invisible laser composed of neodynium ions in an Yttrium-Aluminum-Garnet, thus, officially, Nd:YAG

eye gradually evolved from "oh, God how am I going to do this one?" to a fairly-positive-but-still-not-sure, "I know it is done." Then, finally, I knew the solution would appear, and, it quickly did. In cyberspace, of course. What better place to find it than that non-reality reality, that non-physical space called the Internet!

Following a thread in a forum on eye floaters like mine, I arrived at *eyefloaters.com*, a website created by a scientist and ophthalmologist in Virginia who had solved several problems inherent with the use of lasers for eradicating floaters, with a series of inventions he'd patented and was now just beginning to use in practice. Not only was he an innovator in the field, he was doing a research study under the US Food and Drug Administration on laser eradication of just the kind of floaters, um, *intraocular opacities*, I had. And if that weren't enough, he was a ham radio operator like me! Egads, what more did I need to know?!!

I found his e-mail address and sent him a note, "ham to ham." I said I was intrigued by his work, but nervous. (A friend once told me "Don't ever let doctors mess with your spherical organs!" Well I'd already done that once, so…) He fired back a courteous and detailed description of what he did and how he did it and why it worked. He offered letters from others (other hams, even!) who had already had the treatment. I read them and queried the authors. They were unanimously and unequivocally positive about their results. The doctor was in suburban Washington, DC. I scheduled an appointment.

But the question kept gnawing at the base of my sub-conscious, "How could I tell others to talk to their bodies when I had to go to a 'meat doctor' again?" And I cancelled the first appointment. Oh, I know, I believed everything I have said about the universality of our existence, etc., etc., etc., but when it came right down to it, I didn't want to have to have outside help, I wanted to do it *by myself* (sound like some children you've known?).

First mistake, again. When will I ever learn? It's never necessary to do it alone. "No man is an island." Accept the help from whatever part of your universe, your reality, your world, it comes. If it works, use it.

The second mistake was that I didn't realize what I really needed to do. When I finally decided to keep the next appointment, I thought I was just going to go into this man's office and give myself up to his hands. ("Doctor," remember? White coat, *powerful father* image.) It didn't work that way.

I flew to Washington and checked into a hotel near his office. Next morning at the appointed time I shook hands with the great doctor, handed him one of my "QSL" cards (the traditional information cards hams exchange to confirm their radio contacts), and put myself in his proficient hands. He dilated my eyes, inspected them, and said, "I see why you're here. That's a pretty good sized Weiss ring. Well, no problem, we'll have that thing gone in no time."

But that wasn't the way it would turn out. That "thing" was going to become a big, nearly insurmountable problem.

Wasting no time, after a thorough inspection of my eyes, he scheduled the first laser session for right after lunch – it would take a couple times to get everything – then, driving with my dilated eyes like an old man with cataracts and thick glasses, I nursed my rental car a few blocks down the street to a restaurant for lunch. I was elated, it would soon be over. I wasn't thinking about talking to my body any longer, I was thinking about this genius taking target practice on my eye.

I returned after lunch, and we moved into the command room. He positioned me in the chair and turned on his space age gun. I leaned forward, and locked my chin and forehead into the braces to give him a steady target. "Close your teeth together," he admonished, "and open both eyes." He needed a steady target and a clear field of fire. Then he positioned the magical lens he had invented onto my eye, and readied himself to commence firing. Leaning forward, he looked through the eyepiece of the laser and into the interior of my eye. I saw the bright white light illuminating the inside of my eye, and the red aiming light of the laser. It felt like I was standing behind the target at a firing range.

I waited for the first shot, but nothing happened. He just kept looking with the powerful lens. He moved the laser around, as if seeking a better angle to shoot from. He had me look left, right, up, down. He still didn't shoot.

Then he said, "I have some bad news." I don't think I'm going to be able to get that big guy after all." I couldn't believe my ears. He had been so confident a couple hours ago. "Why?" I asked, almost choking.

"That ring is much farther back in the eye than I thought it was. With this lens, I can see exactly where it is, and it's too close to the retina and the optic nerve to chance shooting at. The laser beam will hit it and scatter, and still have enough power to damage the retina. These things have to be farther away from the retina before I can shoot them. Yours is too close. It's too dangerous."

I said nothing, but leaned harder into the braces holding my head.

"I'm going to go get two of the smaller ones, and then we'll take another look at the ring, but I don't think I'm going to be able to do anything with it."

"Sure," I said, any vestige of hope gone from my soul.

He proceeded to shoot off 50 or so rounds of red-line ammo at a few not-very bothersome floaters, destroying them easily. I watched from behind the target as each noisy "crack" in my head caused another piece of something to detach and float down out of my field of vision.[23] When he'd miss, there would be the click of his footswitch firing the laser, but no "crack." He missed only a couple times, but he wasn't shooting toward the retina anyway, so it didn't matter.

Finally he stopped, and said, "Okay, I got those. Let me take another look at the big one. He had me move my eye, and he repositioned the laser and the lens. Time and time again he'd try a new angle, but never took a shot. Then he fired twice, "crack, crack," and then turned off the laser and flipped on the overhead room lights. He leaned back on his stool, and I did the same on mine. He shook his head.

"I know that this is why you flew all the way here from California," he said, "and I'm really sorry to have to tell you that I just can't get at it. It's not going to be possible to get that one. I'd wind up damaging your retina, and you could lose some of your vision. We can't do that."

He led me back into the examining room. I was practically dragging my feet, like a 6-year old whose daddy had told him he was going to take him to a baseball game, but then announced he had to work, instead. How can this be? I wondered.

But those words once again echoed in my brain: "We can't do that." And almost without thinking, I said, "Listen, if I come back tomorrow and we try again, what are the chances it might be in a better position so you can hit is with the laser? Two percent?" He shrugged, "I don't know." I continued, emboldened by past experience, "…'cause if it's two percent, I'll take it. I'm Mister Two Percent, you know. Let's give it another try tomorrow, maybe I can get it into the right position for you. I'll work with you, we'll get it." I said the words, but my heart wasn't in them.

Neither was his. "I'm really sorry," he said.

---

[23] The doctor corrected me: What I saw floating "down" were actually gas bubbles (from the laser vaporizing the floater) going <u>upward</u>! Remember, the brain flips the image, so I saw them as falling down.

I had to come back tomorrow anyway, for him to check out the other eye while I was there, and look again at the right eye to see what else he ought to get out. It was the normal procedure, to come back the second day, even though I was really only there for that one thing, the big Weiss ring. Any other minor things that might be floating around in my eye my brain would ignore, like most of us do.

The doctor led me into the waiting room, where I put on a game face for the other patients. One asked me how it went, and I said "Well, we got a good start. We're going to get the rest of it tomorrow." But I didn't believe it.

It was raining outside when I walked to the car. Some tropical storm was heading up the Carolina coast and throwing water out of the sky all the way up to the suburbs of Washington, DC, where I was. It was fitting. It was, after all, that part of the movie where the hero's always the most depressed, and the script calls for rain to emphasize the point, just in case you haven't gotten it already.

I drove back to the hotel, and on the way my wife called on the cell phone from home. "I figured I'd catch you just about done with the first session. I couldn't wait for you to call me; how'd it go?" You don't mince words with your best friend, and I told her everything that had happened. Her reply was quick and to the point. "Well you can fix that!" I said I hoped so. I was going back to the hotel room to try. "Oh, don't worry, honey, you'll get it," she said, and I believed she believed it.

As for me, I wasn't that sure. Doctors are powerful people; we hang on their words and opinions about our health. They seriously affect our outlook on our lives. The Doctor had said he couldn't do it. Who was I to believe otherwise?

Then fear struck me. What if he couldn't get the floater? How could I possibly tell people about my process of healing if I couldn't even do this simple thing? I was about to fail. I imagined returning home, and living with that big ring in my eye. I knew I couldn't consider telling people to talk to their bodies when I had that thing I could not deal with. Physician, heal thyself!

Then I realized, I *hadn't* failed at this. In fact, I hadn't done anything. I had not participated with the doctor, I had simply put myself into his hands and become his patient, period. But he could only do what he could do. If he couldn't hit the floater for fear of damaging the retina, maybe I needed to get involved. Maybe I really could help the floater find a better position. It was, after all, *possible*! Clearly if this was going to work, I was going to have to participate, too.

Now I knew why this was unfolding this way: He wasn't going to do it, WE were going to do it. I had to get to work.

In my hotel room I put the "do not disturb" sign on the door, took off my shoes, and crawled up onto the bed. I crossed my legs, and considered trying to sit in the lotus position, I've always wanted to do that, but have always found it too cramped and confining, so I just crossed my legs and leaned over until my elbows rested on the bed. And then I started to moan. Unlike many who meditate, I seem to only use half of that favorite chant "Om," just the clear, throaty "ohhhh" of a good moan. It unloads the emotions.

This was the moment of truth. I needed freedom, hope, belief, clarity, knowingness. I had none of those at the moment. After letting out my feelings, I went back to the rudiments of my process, and started counting down from three like I had learned so many years ago. I descended deep into the inner rooms I had created in my mind those many years ago, and slipped into my eye next to the big ring suspended next to my retina.

"Why are you here?" I asked it, then didn't wait for an answer. "I love you" (I didn't), I continued, "I know you came into my life for a reason, and I thank you, but now it's okay to leave. You may go back through the doorway into energy, into God, it's really okay." I waited. That didn't seem to be getting me anywhere, so I changed tactics (it's always a creative dance). "Okay, is there something else I'm supposed to know before you leave? I'm here. Talk to me."

The emotion hit me before the thought did, but the thought was powerful. These Biblical verses of Matthew floated into my mind[24]:

> *"And why beholdest thou the mote that is in thy brother's eye, but consider not the beam that is in thine own eye? Or how wilt thou say to thy brother, Let me pull out the mote out of thine eye; and, behold, a beam is in thine own eye? Thou hypocrite, first cast out the beam out of thine own eye; and then shalt thou see clearly to cast out the mote out of thy brother's eye.*

I did not hear those words, I never "hear" these things, but the awareness of that passage came clear to me, and the words "first cast the beam out of thine own eye," which I had heard in so many fire-brimmed sermons as a child, struck me hard. So did "thou hypocrite."

What was I doing? Writing a book about how to help your body heal, when there was this big thing in my eye that I couldn't even get out. What a hypocrite! How could I possibly tell others how to take the "mote" out of their own eyes when I couldn't get the "beam" out of mine.

Just as obviously, that passage also relates to judgment of others. And I knew it. No matter how long you dodge an issue, life's going to throw it up in your face again and again, until you deal with it finally. I remembered the Peace Pilgrim, and a thousand other instances of quick and unfair judgment I had cast

---

[24] Since my formative years were spent with the Bible as spiritual guide, my moments of truth often come wrapped in Biblical sayings. Yours will no doubt emerge from your own spiritual heritage.

on people in my life. How many times in my life had I harshly judged someone, and then felt guilty for it, realized I'm the last person who should be judging others, and then gone and done it again. Over the years I had gotten better, perhaps, but certainly not free from heavy-handed judgment. Now here, in this hotel room in Virginia, it was confronting me again. How ironic. How perfect. How just like life, the universe, God, to keep giving you something over and over in different ways until you finally face it. We can never run from anything, can we?

There in the room, I felt I knew what the message was to me: if I didn't own up now to a life of painful judgmentalness, I might lose the chance to get this beam out of my eye, literally.

During the next hour I sat there on the bed, in that state of in-between, conscious only of the dialogue between the Universe and me – God and me – and the beam in my eye and me. My part of the dialogue was aloud, as always. This time it was mostly "I understand," and, "I see" (ironically). And of course "Thank you," is always a big part.

For me, there is always a vestige of my childhood religion in those moments. When I'm deep in the experience of the moment, I like to rock back and forth, to feel my body sway, just like the saints from my old church did when they were "dwelling in the spirit." The first thing they would do would be "lay their troubles down on the altar," and then open themselves to God. They knew they couldn't "pray through" if they were still hanging on to something. Likewise, when you're looking for healing and you talk to your body and it tells you there's something you need to deal with, you'd better deal with it, or healing will elude you.

I remember the story of a man who had throat cancer, and it only went into remission after he underwent intense psychotherapy, during which he remembered stabbing his sister in the neck when they were very young. He had never forgiven himself for that, until that moment. But when he did, he soon discovered his cancer was gone.

Remember, we are body, mind and spirit, the grand trinity all right inside us. When one is affected, the other two know it, and show it. In my experience often a physical illness is the manifestation of a problem in one of the other parts of our reality. So sometimes we have to "lay our burdens down" and get forgiveness. Acknowledging the problem is the first step. Accepting forgiveness is the second – for forgiveness is always at hand. Forgiving yourself is often the hardest part.

So I spent some time there on the bed making a commitment, to paraphrase those old faith healers, to "leave my judgmental nature right there in that room." It was only then that I began to believe I could have a meaningful dialogue with the floater. Only then did it seem to begin to listen to me.

And then I was able to assume of the role of captain of my ship once again. But what should I say to my new friend? In this case, I decided "go to the light" was pretty appropriate. The Light. Aren't words wonderful! "Tomorrow, friend, when you see the red light, go to it. It's coming to take you home to God. You've done your job here, and I am grateful. This is exactly what should happen, it's what I want, and it's perfect. Go to the light, my friend." That's what I said. And I said it aloud, over and over, until I believed, no, I *knew* it would happen.

Then I gave great thanks for all that had happened, "was done," (already accomplished) and then slowly floated up and out of my deep state and looked out the window at the beautiful rain. And just at that moment, the telephone rang. Perfect, I thought. Absolutely perfect. It was a friend, asking about dinner plans that evening. I promptly forgot about everything that had just taken place, but now I knew tomorrow was going to be successful.

Letting go completely is the last step.

The next morning I woke up to rain again. That tropical depression was still out there, but now it was a pleasant, soothing rain. Over breakfast I tried to think of what words to use about the (already accomplished) success with the ring. You may remember at times like this I always like to speak of the future as if it is already done. What first kept coming to mind were variations of "I can't believe he got it so easily," and "I can't believe it just disappeared," but I didn't like the use of "I can't believe." Part of me thinks that at this level maybe our minds are pretty simplistic and might misunderstand the words; hearing and applying the literal meaning "I can not believe," instead of the reverse meaning our idiomatic use of our language gives them. So I chose "It's amazing how easily he was able to completely obliterate it." And I decided to say that aloud as I dressed and drove to the doctor's office.

But suddenly I realized I was going to have to tell the doctor, too. I had to, in order to become a partner in the process. Otherwise I might sink back to the powerless doctor-patient role. And that wouldn't work, we'd already tried that. I was scared again. I'd never done anything like this in my life.

Yet I was clear there was no choice. This was my moment, and I wasn't going to screw it up. I sat in the waiting room rehearsing just what I was going to say, but before I got anything figured out that felt comfortable, the door opened and he called my name.

As I entered the exam room, I opened my mouth to speak but he spoke first. "Let's just begin by looking at your other eye, and make sure there's nothing there we should take care of while you're here. Then we'll take one more look at your right eye and see what's what, but…"

I interrupted him. "Before we begin, I need two minutes of your time. I have to tell you a story," "Okay," he said, curiously, and sat down on his stool.

"I have to tell you that I'm a healer," I blurted out. I didn't mean to say that, but out it came. "I don't mean I heal other people, I mean I heal myself." And then I proceeded to go into a hodgepodge of my history, starting with my background in a faith healing religion and ending up with the story about my macular pucker 18 years ago. "They gave me a two percent chance to have any vision in my right eye in five months, and now it's 18 years later and you yourself tested me at 20/25 vision in both eyes." He nodded in agreement.

"Did you see any sign of a macular pucker?"

"No."

"So I tell you that we don't know the future, and it is possible that when you and I go into that treatment room together, working together we will get that Weiss ring out of my eye. Even if there's only a two percent chance, it is possible. Do you agree?"

He hemmed a bit, and said, "Yes, I agree, it is possible."

"Then let's go in there together, and I will work with you, doing my part inside my body, and somehow magically that ring will move away from the retina enough for you to hit it safely with the laser. Okay?"

"That would be great," he answered.

"I create the possibility…that's what I like to say…I create that it's done." I shrugged now, and sat down in the examining chair. Probably the scariest speech I ever gave since that night I asked my wife to marry me.

But I had just made myself a partner in the endeavor. Together we were going to obliterate the ring. I knew it. He didn't, yet, but it was enough for me that he accepted the possibility that it could happen, and he had done that.

We then proceeded to follow his plan. He examined my left eye, saw a few things he could zap while I was there, and then looked again at my right eye. He didn't spend much time on it, though, saying that he'd have a real look at it with the more accurate laser lens in the treatment room. We moved there.

Adjusting the stool, numbing my eye, placing my chin and forehead in the braces, bringing the laser into position, putting the special lens over my cornea. Ready. Using his laser and lens, a medical miracle all by itself, he shot the left eye first, annihilating little vitreous collagen strands I hadn't really paid much attention to because of the big thing in my right eye. Easy, and successful. He took out the lens, leaned back, turned on the overhead lights, cleaned the lens and my eye, and said, "Okay, let's look at that right eye."

I blurted out once again, "It is possible that you're going to be able to get it." Trying to find a common spiritual language between us, I said, "God works in mysterious ways. Miracles happen." He agreed, but didn't hold out much hope. "You're going to be amazed," I said, with as much confidence as I could possibly muster. "You just tell me where you want me to put it, and I'll get it to go there."

He put the aiming lens in my right eye, repositioned the laser and turned off the lights. "Okay, let's see what we can do." And just like the day before, he moved the lens around looking for a clean shot. For my part, I'd gone deep into my eye again, silently (this time) reminding that clump of collagen to "go to the light" and saying to myself, "It's amazing how easily it's working." I said these two things over and over, breaking only to say aloud to the doctor, "Where do you need me to put it? I'll fling that thing anywhere you want, just tell me."

"Look left." I did. "Look back to center." I did. When I did this, the ring floated into a different position in my eye for a moment. As it did, he looked for a clean shot. Nothing. "Look right." I did. "Look center." Nothing.

In spite of no evidence, yet, I continued my internal celebration of it having been successfully done, and my encouragement of the ring to go to the light, the strong white light of his scope, or the sharp red light of the laser's aiming beam. I imagined I was standing alongside the ring, coaxing it forward with my hands, "Go ahead, it's all right, go."

"Look up." I did. "Look center." Remembering that occasionally I could sling the thing out of my field of vision by moving my eye sharply from one position to another, this time I jerked my eye from top to center quickly, and stopped it there. "Wait, hold it," he said. Crack! He took a shot. Crack, crack, crack, three more hits. "Do that again." I did, and once again he hit it four quick times with the laser. "I can't believe it," he said, "you're moving it away from the retina." On the brace, my teeth were clenched hard so as to not move my head one millimeter, but inside my head I was screaming "Yay! It's amazing how easily he's getting it! It's done! He got the whole thing!" while outside I was listening to the tenor of his voice and breathing, looking for any hint one way or the other.

We hung on there together as he directed the movement of my eye, and each time I moved it, the slowly disintegrating ring would slide up and away from the retina just enough for him to hit it again with the laser. "It's no longer a ring, now," he said, "it's a C." More eye moves, more cracks of laser hitting collagen. Inside my eye I could not see the hit – I dare not see that – but after each hit I could see once again what looked like little pieces of the thing falling away from the center of my eye.

More laser hits, constantly supported by my internal "It's just amazing how easily this thing is disappearing!" The sharpshooter didn't speak for awhile, intent on his work. When he did, he said "You are the luckiest person I've ever seen, I've got about 50% of this thing!" My left eye started to cry, and my heart gushed with appreciation. My "It's amazing just how easily..." chant was now filled with absolute joy.

Soon he announced he had 80%, and then 98%, and he stopped. "I know from experience, this is when you can run into trouble," he said, and I didn't push it. There was a follow-up session already scheduled for the next morning, and I figured he could clean out the rest then.

He turned off the laser, took out the lens and flipped on the lights. We looked at each other, and smiled. "I would never have believed it," he said, and shook his head. "You actually made that thing move away from the retina, just enough that I could safely hit it. I've never seen that before."

Twenty-five years ago I met the renowned cancer doctor Gerald Jampolski, a friend of a friend who ran into each other in a San Francisco restaurant. When we said goodbye I reached out to shake his hand but instead he hugged me – in public! A big, comfortable bear hug – the first time a stranger had ever done that. Seeing my discomfort, he told me "Five hugs a day! It's the greatest gift you can give another person."

In that simple ground-floor office in a nondescript building in this Washington suburb, I stood up from the magical laser, wiped my eyes, and hugged this genius inventor, this human being, who had taken a step with me into faith that he had never taken before. Our faith together had left me with a clear eye, where yesterday it had not been possible.

"You're one in a million," he said.

No, I just act on my beliefs.

You can, too.

Ten years later Dr. John Karickhoff, ophthalmologist and inventor, still uses the procedure we created together on many of his patients. He calls it "the Moses Maneuver."

I don't know how well I will do at never being judgmental again. Every time I hit the freeway at rush hour I still want to be Traffic Cop. Probably next time someone new shows up at church in an orange Mohawk and Doc Martin boots I'll cringe again. But I know there is only one way to absolutely perfect health, and that's through perfect release of guilt, fear, frustration, anger…and my two favorites, avarice and greed, however you find it possible to achieve. It may never be absolutely possible, but we can keep working on it.

One way to start is with that long-overdue dialogue with your best friend, your body. It has so much it wants to tell you about yourself.

APPENDIX

HOW TO TALK TO YOUR BODY
(The Long Way)

Step 1: **First Relax**

Step 2: **Explore, Create, Imagine**

Step 3: **Listen, Apologize, Be Honest**

Step 4: **Repair, Physically and Psychologically**

Step 5: **Insist, Love, Cajole, Coach**

Step 6: **Give Thanks**

Step 7: **Release and Know**

Step 8: **Now Go Do Something Else Fun**

Read through the following first, before trying it. **If you want to read this into a recorder to play back to yourself as a guide, read only the words in boldface type.** The rest is explanatory only.

Step 1: Relax

You are the Captain, be not afraid.

Find a private place to sit or lie down where you can stay for some length of time without becoming uncomfortable. You can even do it while running or walking, so long as it won't bother you knowing that there might be other people listening to you. However you relax, relax, and close your eyes.

Now we're going to start the process of moving into that black period of our reality. It should be a fun imaginary experience, but at first it may be a little disorienting, or even scary. Don't worry, you're never alone. You're imagining everything you think and do, and it's all under your direct control at all times. If it becomes too much, just stop, open your eyes, and go get a beer or something. This should be fun, stay light. (Maybe a *light* beer?)

Step 2: Explore, Create, Imagine

If you know how to meditate, start that process, and go into the place where you normally go. If you typically go "to the light," stop before you begin that, and join the process as we enter the "0" below.

If you don't know how to meditate, try this:

After you're comfortable and relaxed, close your eyes and imagine you've drifted into an empty, dark space in your head. You look around and see that you're actually in space, there are stars all around you, and you can see the circles of the paths of the planets. Everything is moving slowly, as in a slow and graceful dance. As you watch this "dance of the spheres," you begin to see in the distance an object moving toward you. As it approaches, slowly and gracefully, turning slowly on itself, you see that it is the number 3.

As you watch the 3 glide closer to you, notice all the detail about it. See if the sides are smooth or rough, shiny or dull, metal, wood, plastic, whatever they are, notice it, as it moves toward you. Then notice that it is three-dimensional, and look at the way the number is formed. However it appears, take a thorough look at it.)

As it moves quite close to you now, you will see that it is very big, much bigger than you are, and that it has a hole through it easily big enough for you to glide through. Make yourself smaller if you like, and swim through the hole in the 3 as if you're gliding underwater through a beautiful cave. Notice as you go what the inside of the hole looks like, and then flip your fins and cruise on out the other side, into the beautiful blackness of space once again.

Enjoy the view of the stars and the rings of the planets' paths, maybe you'll see a few shooting stars while you're there, but then notice in the distance another objecting moving toward you. As it draws near, you see it is the number 2, just like the 3 before. As it approaches, notice all the detail about it. See what shape of 2 it is.

(Look at the sides, and see how the pieces are joined together. Maybe this is the works of a lone carver, or maybe it is has been extruded from a mold. Maybe it is nickel, or titanium, or stainless steel that has been welded together. Or maybe it's made out of leaves and grass, like a thatched roof. Whatever you see, see it clearly, and in great detail.)

Now as the 2 moves close to you, and you see how large it is, notice that there is a hole in its side, too. As before with the 3, glide through the hole, and out the other side into space once again. Enjoy the comfortable trip.

Now in the distance is the 1, moving slowly toward you. Observe it as you have the others, then as it is close, see the hole and glide through it out to the other side.

Now you will see a formless place, an opening to somewhere else. The shape of the opening is the number 0, and you are moving toward it slowly and gracefully. As you approach the 0, you move through its center, and descend slowly down into an elevator, your personal elevator, which has been waiting for you.

(Look at the elevator in detail. Is it a small French style elevator, with wrought iron filigree everywhere, or is it a sleek elevator found in modern office buildings? Or maybe it's an industrial elevator, with a rope to close the double doors. Whatever you see, that's your elevator.)

Close the doors, if that's necessary, and then you will notice on the side wall the number 9. The elevator will begin to descend under your control, from 9 to 8 and so on down to 1. As it does, be sure to clearly see the numbers as they go by. If you can't, slow down the elevator until you do see the number, then descend to the next number, until you reach 1.

The elevator will stop at 1. Get out, leaving the door open if you wish. As you step out of the elevator, you will find yourself in a room with hallways leading in various directions out of it. Look around it, see how it is laid out and decorated. Take a look at a few of the hallways, but don't go down any of them yet.

This is your launching center. From here you can travel to any part of your body at will. Each hallway is actually a nerve pathway which will lead you to whatever area of your body you want to go to. One leads down to the heart and lungs, another out the shoulders, down the arms and into the tips of each finger. Yet another pathway will take you to the abdomen, or genitals, or down your legs to your knees and feet.

There's a pathway from here to every point in your body, and you never get lost. All you have to do is decide that the hallway on your left, for example, leads you down your spinal cord to the back of your right leg where there's a cramp, and you slide down it...

(maybe even going "wheeeee")

...and drop off exactly where the cells or muscles are that you need to talk to.

So now let's do that. Pick a place in your body that has been giving you trouble, and select the pathway out of your room that will take you there. Hook yourself on to the nerve with a safety line, and slide into the tunnel. Ride the nerve (or artery or vein, if you wish) down to the location and step off to greet your crew.

Step 3. Listen, Apologize, Be Honest

When you arrive, remember to be completely honest. You are the captain, and maybe they're looking for succor in their time of fear and trouble, or maybe they just need a good pep talk. You will be able to tell.

(Whatever you determine after you've been there a few minutes will be correct. Remember, there is no wrong way to do this. You are the creator of this experience.)

Just as you carefully observed – visualized – the numbers earlier, and saw the detail in your launch room, now look at the cells and organs, muscles or bones, etc., that you have come to see. However you see them is okay, just make sure you see and sense what they look like.

Now begin a dialogue with them, as if they are your good and faithful friends, and you've come to check up on them and get reacquainted. And, if they are angry or afraid, you're there to make things right. Again, talk out loud, and imagine what they are saying back to you.

(It can – and probably will – be an inane conversation.)

Have the dialogue, listen to it, *but do not edit what is being said.* Let your imagination fly, carry on as if you and they were old drinking buddies.

(What I usually hear is, "It's about time you got down here.")

Step 4: Repair, Physically and Psychologically

Whatever you experience there, act on it, now. If they need help, give them help. If they need fixing, you've got all the tools in your back pocket that you need to fix them right then and there. If they need a hug, give them several. And if they need to let off steam, you're all ears. If they need you to apologize for neglecting them, do it, from the bottom of your heart. And mean it when you say you won't do that again.

Step 5: Insist, Love, Cajole, Coach

Imagine what you would say if you were the coach of a football team that was getting creamed out there on the field, and you had ignored the game and walked into the locker room to make a phone call. Now you're back, and they have needed you. Be there for them. Be the coach – be the captain of the ship. Whatever love and encouragement they need, give it to them, they trust you.

Step 6: Give Thanks

Spend as much time with your crew as you need, until you completely understand that all is well between you, and they are comfortable going back to their perfect function.

Then thank them for the wonderful job they do for you, and say goodbye, promising to always be there for them, and frequently in touch. Let them know they can always count on you from now on, now that you know that you can communicate with them like this.

As you leave them to return to their perfect functioning, know that it's done, and give thanks also to that which created you for the knowledge you have, and for the new reality of a perfectly functioning body. Then you may move to another part of your body, or slowly return to the launch room, greeting other parts of your crew as you move by them, stopping if you wish, to chat and thank them for their excellent work – out loud.

Step 7: Release and Know

Once you have returned to your launch room, look around it again, seeing once again just where everything is,

(decorate it with anything you wish on your next trip),

then turn out the lights if you wish, and step into your elevator.

Ride the elevator back up to the top, and step out into your starry space again. Now, as you look around, you will realize that this space is actually the inside of the medulla oblongata of your brain – the part that connects the brain to the spinal cord. All you need do now is expand your awareness to fill out your brain completely, and you're back home. You can stay there for awhile if you want to, noticing how it feels. Then you may open your eyes whenever you wish.

Now forget everything that just happened, and go do something else.

(It can help to say aloud, "It's done, and I release it to be.")

Step 8: Now Go Do Something Else Fun

It's important to remember to go play.

This entire process works best when it's approached as play, especially the dialogue with your body. Friends play together. If you see something that could mean illness, treat it like it's no more than a bothersome "irregularity" in the cells and wash it away with a rag, or pull out some oil from your back pocket and lubricate it, or whatever you playfully feel it needs, playfully give it. And it's done.

Most of all, don't expect any immediate change. You might, on occasion, feel differently afterward, but usually noticeable changes take some time, especially in the beginning. It's almost as if the universe is testing us, to see if we really accept this, or we're demanding immediate results or we want our money back. Don't look for immediate results. KNOW that it is done, *in the face of no evidence.*

Well, there you are. Those are the rudiments of the full process. Obviously, as you play with it over time, it will become easier, and faster. Soon you won't have to do the entire counting thing, you'll just jump down to whatever hurts, see yourself standing beside it, tools in hand, and start to talk. But you see from my own experiences that too often we forget to use it, even when we know perfectly well how.

THE SHORT WAY

Quickie phrases that work for me

For bumps, scrapes, cuts and other painful would-be injuries: *"Not a word of truth to it,"* followed by a quick trip inside the injury to tell the cells: "Hey you guys, bet that scared you, didn't it? Well, you're fine, everything's just fine..." etc.

For potentially larger problems: *"I am perfect health. I know that my (leg, arm, etc.) is fine. I thought I was injured but I was just mistaken..."* followed by the process.

I suppose you can just go out and play with these things without understanding the fundamentals behind them. Only time will tell, as people begin to experiment and report what they are finding. I would like to hear your stories using these techniques. As we talk to our bodies more and more, we will gain more insights into even better methods than I describe here.

After awhile, perhaps, the "hundredth monkey" effect might even occur, where people will innately know how to do this without ever being taught.

Or maybe that's how we started millions of years ago, and we're just now crawling out of our caves once again to the light.

To the Light?

◊ ◊ ◊

Made in United States
North Haven, CT
20 November 2022